THE LOW-FAT GOURMET

By the same author

Living with Multiple Sclerosis
Grow Your Own Health (*with Keith Mossman*)
Asthma, Hay Fever and Other Allergies

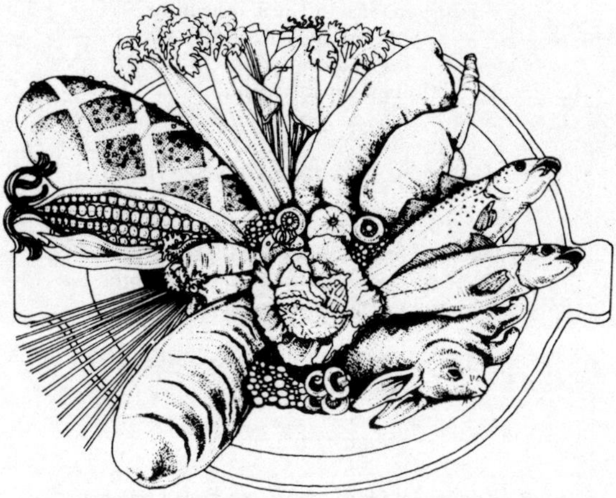

THE LOW-FAT GOURMET

A Doctor's Cookbook for Heart Disease and MS

Dr Elizabeth Forsythe

PELHAM BOOKS
LONDON

First published in Great Britain by
PELHAM BOOKS LTD
44 Bedford Square
London WC1B 3DU
1980

ISBN 0 7207 1226 2

Filmset by Northumberland Press Ltd, Gateshead, Tyne and Wear
Printed in Great Britain by
Billings & Son, Guildford, Surrey

Illustrations by Susan Neale

Contents

Preface

In recent years research work has been carried out on the effects of diet on certain illnesses, including coronary heart disease (CHD) and multiple sclerosis (MS). In both conditions it has been suggested that a diet low in fats will be beneficial and it is on this supposition that this book is written.

Coronary heart disease is commoner in men than in women and is the commonest cause of death in men over thirty-five years of age. It is increasing in extent. Multiple sclerosis is a common disease of the nervous system in temperate climates. It is estimated that there are 50,000 people with MS in the United Kingdom and 250,000 in the United States. Both diseases, therefore, present a widespread and in different ways serious threat to health.

There is no certain way known of preventing CHD or of treating MS. Both diseases probably have a number of causes which may be called multi-factorial. CHD may be started by stress, lack of exercise, overweight and smoking cigarettes; the last factor is probably of the greatest importance. However, there has also been much interest in diet. It is now generally agreed that a reduction in the total amount of fat in the diet is of benefit. At times it has been suggested that certain foods rich in cholesterol should be avoided, but it is now thought that the best way of keeping down the level of cholesterol in the blood is by keeping the fat intake low. It is also thought that animal fats in the diet should be reduced more than other types of fat.

Although there is no known cure for MS, a positive approach to the management of the illness is of inestimable value to the patient and his or her family. Diet is amongst the accepted lines of management and at different times, different diets have been in vogue. There have been one or two dramatic accounts of the effects of a gluten-free diet and a trial was done on a number of patients; no benefit was found and the diet will not be mentioned again in this book. Studies of the incidence of MS have shown it to be more common where a greater amount of animal fat is eaten and less common where oil is eaten. A diet low in animal fat is now frequently recommended.

If you are going to take the diet seriously and you realise you may have to live with it for a great number of years, you may as well learn to live with it happily and graciously. Food should be one of life's pleasures whether you are on a diet or not; and if you are on a diet I think you just have to make an extra effort to make your food a pleasure. It is both time-consuming, more expensive and inelegant to cook and serve different foods for different members of the family. With a few adaptations in materials and in methods of cooking, excellent appetising food which is decidedly acceptable for all members of the family can be cooked and served to all those present for a meal. Nobody in the family will suffer; in fact it is possible that they may benefit from a low-fat diet and the patient will have the security of knowing that he or she is eating what is best for him or her. Being on a diet does not mean putting up with dull food and I hope that the recipes in this book will make that quite clear.

My Credentials for Writing this Book

The first of my credentials for writing this book is that, as a patient with multiple sclerosis, I have now lived on a low-animal-fat diet for more than three years. An unforeseen bonus of this diet is that as long as I stick to it I do not have to worry about counting calories. In fact, there have been times when I have lost too much weight and have had to make a conscious effort to eat more protein and carbohydrate. For every gram of food that the body burns, twice as many calories are produced from fat as from an equal weight of protein or carbohydrate. Up to a point it is: 'Look after the fat and the weight will look after itself.'

I also happen to be a qualified and practising medical practitioner and, partly because of my own illness, have developed a keen interest in nutrition. The low-fat diet has become an incentive to make food more interesting rather than becoming resigned to a loss of pleasure in it. I make no secret of my enjoyment of eating good food whether somebody else has cooked it or whether I have cooked it myself. Perhaps weight would have been less of a problem if I had been one of those women who 'could never eat anything I had prepared' – but I enjoy reading about food, thinking about food, preparing food and eating it! I have a food-conscious husband and three adolescent children who also enjoy meals and who can all be constructively critical as well as appreciative: they are a pleasure to cook for. I have realised that it is impractical to prepare and eat two different meals at once, and it has become quite apparent that it is very much more practical and less tiring to prepare one meal that fits in with any diet and is enjoyed by the entire family. I solved this problem in various ways, including the substitution of sunflower-seed oil for all oil used in the preparation of food. I am not even sure if the family knows this and there has never been an adverse comment. I never use lard, which of course is animal fat, but prepare casseroles, curries, soups, sauces and French dressing with sunflower-seed oil.

The preparations for and the writing of this book have become very much a family affair. All of the recipes have been tested by my family: some have been given a very poor reception and have been altered or rejected. I feel strongly that food and cooking and eating should be a family interest and all of these should be a pleasure. I do not believe that 'gourmet' cooking should be different from family cooking. Even when the young are going through the 'chips, baked beans and fish fingers' stage I think that there should be more sophisticated eating patterns available for when their tastes change.

I have had very little training in cooking but my husband avows that a short intensive course I did at the Cordon Bleu Cookery School in London soon after our marriage was the best-spent period of my life; perhaps he is right. My interest in cooking has been stimulated by my husband's cosmopolitan tastes in eating developed by many years living abroad and also by the fairly extensive travelling which we have done together.

I make no apology for the Scottish bias which creeps repeatedly into the recipes. Having been married to a Scot for a quarter of a century and having lived since 1973 in the far north of Scotland, I have had a good grounding in the best of Scottish cooking and baking. Scottish food is not primarily porridge, herrings and scones; although all of these are excellent. I am fortunate enough to have in my kitchen an 1840 edition of Megg Dodd's Cookery Book. When one is reading that, one is strongly aware of the 'auld alliance' and the influence of French cooking on Scottish.

In trying out recipes, I have of necessity been limited in materials in some directions but have had a very great variety in other ways. Fresh fruit and vegetables can be in short supply in the far north and on occasions I have had to use those that are frozen or tinned. On the other hand I probably find it easier to get fresh fish, venison and hare, all of which are protein foods low in fat. Not many housewives have lobster, crab or a 20-lb turbot left by friends at the back door. I have a ready supply of salt herrings, I can buy the grade of oatmeal that I need and bere meal is ground locally. I am not able to get avocado pears ready for immediate use, nor many other such delicacies.

Preparing and eating food can and, I believe, should be important pleasures in our lives. If you are put on a special diet I think there are good reasons for making the pleasures greater rather than turning your back on them.

About Fats

You really need to know quite a lot about biochemistry to understand the construction of all the individual parts of fat which are called fatty acids. Fat is made up of carbon, hydrogen and oxygen. In the middle of each molecule of any particular fatty acid there is a chain of carbon atoms joined together. If there is a single link between each carbon atom and all the other links available to each carbon atom are taken up by other atoms, the fat is called a saturated fat. If two of the carbon atoms in the central chain are joined together by a double bond while all the rest have single bonds the fat is called a mono-unsaturated fat. If more than two carbon atoms are joined together by double bonds the fat is known as poly-unsaturated fat.

One of the poly-unsaturated fatty acids is linoleic acid and this is called an essential fatty acid; it must be taken in the diet because the body is not able to manufacture it. There is controversial evidence that linoleic acid may help in preventing the damage to nervous tissue in MS. Many doctors encourage their patients to take supplements of linoleic acid either as sunflowerseed (SFS) oil or in capsules. I am advising the use of SFS oil throughout this book when oil is needed in a recipe and sunflowerseed margarine when butter or margarine is necessary.

For the purposes of this book, saturated fats are usually of animal origin. They are solid at room temperature, present in meat and dairy foods and should be curtailed in a diet for a patient with coronary heart disease or multiple sclerosis. It is only possible to put an arbitrary limit on the amount of fat that can be allowed each day and this is usually given as 15g or 3 teaspoons.

Mono-unsaturated and poly-unsaturated fats are usually runny at room temperature, are frequently of vegetable origin and will be called oils throughout this book. It will probably be reasonable to accept a daily intake of 20g or 4 teaspoons as the minimum necessary for health and 50g or 10 teaspoons as the upper limit. It is important that either the total permitted amount of fat should be eaten each day with an adequate amount of oil or, if the fat on any day is reduced, that the amount of oil should be increased. If the total daily intake of fat and oil is reduced too drastically you will become tired, apathetic, possibly depressed and your sleep may be disturbed. Some of these symptoms may occur initially with a low-fat diet in any case, but can usually be relieved by increasing the intake of oil. With time you will become accustomed to the diet and will keep fit on it.

The fat and oil in our diet take longer to digest than the carbohydrate and protein, and they give us a greater feeling of satisfaction after a meal. When your dietary fat and oil are reduced you may find that you are frequently hungry between meals. It is quite permissible to have a snack of skimmed milk and possibly bread with peanut butter which will help top up your oil intake.

It can be a mistake to be too enthusiastic about cutting down on your oils as well as your fats. Each gram of fat burnt by the body produces about 9 calories, each gram of carbohydrate about 4 calories and each gram of protein about 4 calories. I have said 'about' because there are many complicated variations. Without realising it you may be cutting your total daily number of calories too much when you cut down on your fats. Not only will you start to lose weight quite rapidly but you will also be lacking in energy. Weigh yourself each week if you are on this diet and do not allow yourself to become lighter than is a good weight for your height and build.

Each recipe in this book is designed for a family of four but naturally family appetites will vary considerably and at times you will be cooking for more or fewer than four people. At the end of each recipe I give the total amount of fat contained in it and the total amount of oil. Of necessity this will vary quite a lot but it should be fairly easy to work out the approximate amounts for each portion.

If you become less mobile with any disease you will need to take in fewer calories. If you eat more than is necessary for you, you will put on weight; the extra weight will not help your mobility or weak muscles and a vicious circle will be built up. I am not giving the total calories for each recipe because for most people they are irrelevant. If you do need to reduce weight, cut down on sugar and alcohol – particularly spirits; and remember that dry wines contain fewer calories than sweet ones – and in general eat smaller helpings.

A low-animal-fat diet is one which you are going to adopt for life or until medical opinion has changed a great deal. You will not see dramatic results in a month or even in a year, and you will never know how much better you have kept because you have stayed on your diet. I believe that it is a worthwhile positive action to take, and provided your food remains interesting the diet is no hardship. One final piece of advice: remember that, as with any other long-term diet, it is safer to have one big cheat a month than three small cheats every day.

A Table of the Amount of Fat and Oil in Some Commonly Eaten Foods

The measures in the following table are of necessity very approximate. The same food produced in different countries, in different ways and at different times of the year will contain widely varying amounts of fat and oil. To refresh your memory, 'fat' is the word used for saturated fats which are usually set at room temperature. Oil is of mono-unsaturated or poly-unsaturated origin and is liquid at room temperature. In general it is probably best to restrict the daily intake of fat to a maximum of 15g/½oz and of oil to a minimum of 20g/¾oz. Within these limits the possibilities for planning menus are very great.

The table below gives the approximate portion of each food which will contain 5g or 1 teaspoon of fat or oil. The amount of each food will be given in g and oz in the same approximate ratio which is used in the menus throughout the book.

Dairy products such as butter and full-fat cheese contain such large amounts of fat that they must be used very sparingly or banned from the diet. I have used grated Parmesan cheese in small quantities in a number of menus. It is often served separately, and it is easy for the member of the family who is on a low-fat diet to take a very small portion or refrain from eating it altogether.

Ordinary margarine should be treated with the same caution as butter. A special warning must be given about all manufactured foods, including soups, biscuits, cakes and just about any sort of tinned food. There may be a surprisingly large amount of fat 'hidden' in these foods. It is very much better to start your cooking from the raw materials and ban convenience foods from your stores.

FOOD	APPROXIMATE PORTION CONTAINING 5g/1 TEASPOON *FAT*		APPROXIMATE PORTION CONTAINING 5g/1 TEASPOON *OIL*	
Fish	g	oz		
Cod	225	8		
Crab	150	6		
Eel				
smoked	25	1		
Haddock				
fresh	225	8		
smoked	225	8		
Halibut	100	4		
Herring				
fresh	25	1		
pickled	25	1		
smoked	50	2		
Lobster	225	8		
Mackerel				
fresh	50	2		
smoked	50	2		
Mussels	225	8		
Salmon	50	2		
Shrimps	225	8		
Trout	225	8		
Tuna	25	1		

Vegetables

Most vegetables contain minimal amounts of fat and oil and can be eaten in an unlimited quantity provided that fat is not used in their preparation. Chips are banned.

	g	oz	g	oz
Broad beans	225	8		
Soya beans	75	3	50	2

Fruit

Nearly all fruit may be eaten in unlimited quantities because it contains negligible amounts of fat and oil.

	g	oz	g	oz
Avocado pear	225	8	225	8
Olives	50	2		

A Table of the Amount of Fat and Oil in Some Commonly Eaten Foods

FOOD	APPROXIMATE PORTION CONTAINING 5g/1 TEASPOON *FAT*		APPROXIMATE PORTION CONTAINING 5g/1 TEASPOON *OIL*	
Nuts	g	oz		
Almonds	10	½	50	2
Brazils	10	½	25	1
Chestnuts	500	16		
Cashews	10	½	225	8
Hazelnuts	10	½	25	1
Peanuts	25	1	50	2
Walnuts	50	2	10	½
Cereals				
Bread				
pumpernickel	350	12		
white	225	8		
Flour				
buckwheat	225	8		
maize	225	8		
rye	350	12		
white	350	12		
wholemeal	225	8		
Oat flakes	225	8	225	8
Rice				
brown	350	12		
polished	500	16		
Semolina				
maize	350	12		
wheat	500	16		
Wheatgerm	50	2	225	8
Fats				
Butter	*Avoid*			
Cheese				
Cheddar	25	1		
cream	25	1		
Emmental	25	1		
Mozzarella	35	1½		
Parmesan	25	1		
skimmed cottage	225	8		

FOOD	APPROXIMATE PORTION CONTAINING 5g/1 TEASPOON *FAT*		APPROXIMATE PORTION CONTAINING 5g/1 TEASPOON *OIL*	
Eggs				
whole	1 egg		1 egg	
white	Unlimited			
yolk	25g	1oz		
Lard	*Avoid*			
Margarine	*Avoid*			
ordinary				
poly-unsaturated fat (PUF)	25g	1oz	5g	$\frac{1}{4}$oz
Milk				
whole	50ml	2oz		
dried skimmed	Unlimited			
Oil				
corn	*Avoid*			
olive	*Avoid*			
safflower			5g	1 teaspoon
sunflower-seed (SFS)			5g	1 teaspoon
Yoghurt				
commercial low-fat	225g	8oz		
home-made skimmed	Unlimited			
Meat	g	oz		
Bacon, lean	25	1		
Beef, lean	50	2		
Chicken, without skin	100	4		
Ham, lean	25	1		
Hare	225	8		
Heart, lean	75	3		
Kidney	150	6		
Lamb, lean leg	75	3		
Liver	150	6		
Rabbit	150	6		
Turkey, without skin	100	6		
Venison	225	8		

Notes on the Ingredients used in the Recipes

The smoothness and richness of many gourmet dishes may not be achieved with the recipes in this book because of the restrictions on ingredients, such as cream and egg yolks, which provide these qualities. In order to make the food more enjoyable and add to its interest I have concentrated on contrast in both texture and flavour. When planning menus you can carry this contrast throughout a meal and your family may find, as mine has done, great pleasure in new eating habits.

In particular, we have become accustomed to a fairly large individually prepared side salad with meat and fish dishes. We may have cooked vegetables as well, but the enjoyment of cooked vegetables can be marred without the addition of butter which is forbidden. On the other hand, a fresh crisp white cabbage, finely grated and mixed with fruit, is delicious served with a French or fruit-juice dressing made with sunflower-seed oil instead of olive oil.

Home-made rye bread or whole cob bread provides another interesting texture; brown rice and pasta cooked no more than is necessary both give pleasure in biting and tasting. Cheesecakes have become very popular because there is a nice contrast between the crisp base and the soft velvety texture of the upper layer. We find that these contrasts in texture and flavour are adequate compensation for the loss of cream, cheese, butter, egg yolks and whole milk.

Certain meats which are high in animal fat, such as pork and pork products, have been entirely omitted from these recipes and from the table of fat content in various foods on pp. 15–18. It may be surprising that, even when you are eating lean meat, more than half the calories you obtain are from fat and not from protein.

For this reason it is advisable to limit your red meat to two meals a week unless you are able to obtain venison or hare which are both high in protein and very low in fat. Poultry contains less fat if you remove the skin and fish is the most suitable protein food of all, being the lowest in fat – with the exception of herring, mackerel and tinned fish.

Certain high-fat foods associated with 'gourmet' recipes are virtually impossible to replace. There is no reason why you should not have an egg in a recipe, providing the fat in the yolk is counted in your daily total fat intake. Cream is a problem; I find that no fat-free or low-fat substitute is really acceptable and I have tended to follow the new French method of cooking, *Cuisine Minceur*, rather than try to pretend that synthetic cream is real cream. I have, however, used substitutes in some recipes (see pp. 22–6).

Cheese is another problem and Parmesan is irreplacable in so many favourite dishes. In this case, a *small* quantity can be counted in your daily fat allowance. Mozzarella and Jarlsburg are relatively low in fat but should still be used in moderation and an allowance made for their fat content in your total intake for the day. Cottage cheese of the low-fat sort can be used liberally but the high-fat cream cheese should be avoided altogether.

Although it is necessary to curtail the amount of red meat in the diet, the amount of protein eaten should not be restricted. Protein intake may be boosted by the lavish use in cooking of skimmed-milk powder, home-made skimmed-milk yoghurt and also by using unrefined cereals such as wholemeal flour and brown rice whenever possible. Protein-containing vegetables, such as lentils and all variations of beans, are another useful adjunct to the diet. They can be eaten in soups, casseroles, as vegetables, and cold as salads.

In all the recipes in this book dried skimmed milk is used either as powder or made up into its liquid form according to the directions provided with the particular brand. Use a type of milk that has a negligible amount of fat in it, and ensure it has no vegetable fat added. Recipes requiring a small quantity of yoghurt can be made up with a commercial preparation, but if large quantities are needed, home-made skimmed-milk yoghurt should be used.

The oil used in all recipes is sunflower-seed (SFS) oil. It may be bought most economically by the gallon from whole or real food stores. If margarine is necessary, poly-unsaturated fat (PUF) margarine should be used or sunflower-seed margarine if it is available.

I have used alcohol in a number of recipes in this book. There is no reason why it should not be used if you have MS or CHD unless weight control is a problem (in which case, simply omit it from the recipes in which it is included) or, of course, unless you do not enjoy the flavour of alcohol.

All herbs used in the recipes are dried with the exception of parsley and chives. If you wish to substitute fresh herbs, use about twice the volume given for dried.

Home-Made Substitutes used throughout this Book

French Dressing

It is a good idea to make this in fairly large quantities and always have it ready.

45ml/3 tablespoons SFS oil
15ml/1 tablespoon wine vinegar
crushed garlic or other herbs as desired
5ml/1 teaspoon salt

Mix all the ingredients together and stir or shake vigorously. Keep in a cool place.
Fat: Nil
Oil: 60g/12 teaspoons

Lemon or Orange Dressing

A fruit dressing makes a pleasant change from French dressing with delicately flavoured salads.

15ml/1 tablespoon lemon or orange juice
5ml/1 teaspoon sugar
45ml/3 tablespoons SFS oil

Mix all ingredients together and stir or shake vigorously.
Fat: Nil
Oil: 60g/12 teaspoons

Low-Fat Home-Made Yoghurt

For this recipe it is very much easier to use a commercial thermostatically controlled type of yoghurt maker. For starting the mixture you may use 45ml/3 tablespoons of a bought tub of low-fat natural yoghurt, or a packet of the appropriate ferment – in which case you must follow the instructions for preparation – or you can perpetuate your supply by taking 45ml/3 tablespoons of the last batch to start your new batch. It is better to make your own yoghurt if your family enjoys eating it in considerable quantities. All the commercially prepared yoghurt has at least two per cent fat in it. If you are going to use only a tablespoon or two in a recipe the amount of fat is negligible and there is no point in making your own.

75g/3oz powdered skimmed milk
600ml/1 pint warm water
prepared culture or 45ml/3 tablespoons previous batch of yoghurt

Whisk all the ingredients together thoroughly. Put them in your yoghurt maker and leave for about ten hours.
Fat: Nil
Oil: Nil

Sour-Cream Substitute

100g/4oz low-fat cottage cheese
15ml/1 tablespoon skimmed milk
50g/2oz home-made skimmed-milk yoghurt

Blend all the ingredients together in an electric blender until smooth. This recipe is excellent served on soups which would normally need sour cream. It can also be used with salt-herring recipes.
Fat: Nil
Oil: Nil

Mayonnaise Substitute

125g/5oz home-made yoghurt
5ml/1 teaspoon salt
5ml/1 teaspoon French mustard
4 drops Tabasco sauce
5ml/1 teaspoon sugar
30ml/2 tablespoons SFS oil

Blend the yoghurt and mustard in an electric blender. Add the oil very slowly, mixing continuously. Add the other ingredients and blend until evenly mixed.
Fat: Nil
Oil: 40g/8 teaspoons

Mustard Sauce

Mustard sauce keeps well in the refrigerator and is good with beef and ham dishes.

45ml/3 tablespoons made English mustard
15ml/1 tablespoon vinegar
salt to taste
60ml/4 tablespoons apricot jam
125g/5oz home-made yoghurt

Blend the mustard, apricot jam and vinegar in an electric blender until quite smooth. Blend in the yoghurt until evenly distributed and add salt to taste.
Fat: Nil
Oil: Nil

White Sauce

15ml/1 tablespoon PUF margarine
450ml/¾ pint skimmed milk
15ml/1 tablespoon cornflour
salt and pepper

Melt the margarine in a saucepan and stir in the cornflour. Cook over a gentle heat until smooth. Add the milk, stirring all the time, bring to the boil and simmer for one minute. Season to taste.
Fat: 5g/1 teaspoon
Oil: 15g/3 teaspoons

Tomato Sauce

Delicious with kedgeree and other fish dishes.

4 tomatoes
½ wine glass white wine
15ml/1 tablespoon flour
pinch oregano
salt and pepper
1 small onion
15ml/1 tablespoon SFS oil
5ml/1 teaspoon sugar
3ml/½ teaspoon basil
1 bay leaf

Chop the onion finely and remove the tomato skins. Simmer the tomatoes, wine, onion and bay leaf together for about twenty minutes. Remove the bay leaf and pass the mixture through a sieve. Warm the oil, stir in the flour and mix well over a low heat. Add the tomato mixture, herbs and sugar and cook uncovered, stirring continuously until the sauce has thickened. Season to taste.
Fat: Nil
Oil: 20g/4 teaspoons

Cream Substitute

This quantity makes enough for a recipe requiring 100g/4oz cream.

50g/2oz powdered skimmed milk
15ml/1 tablespoon lemon juice
25g/1oz caster sugar
45ml/3 tablespoons cold water
1g/¼ teaspoon powdered gelatine

Dissolve the gelatine in 15ml/1 tablespoon of water over a low heat. Add the other 30ml/2 tablespoons of water to the dried milk, lemon juice and sugar and whisk until of an even consistency. Add the cooled gelatine mixture and whisk again until frothy. Put the mixture in a freezer or the freezer compartment of a refrigerator for about half an hour. Whisk again for about five minutes and then use in a recipe or serve with a dessert. This recipe will not cook but will freeze well.
Fat: Nil
Oil: Nil

Vanilla Sauce for use with Hot Puddings and Fruit

40g/1½oz cornflour
25g/1oz granulated sugar
450ml/¾ pint skimmed milk
few drops vanilla essence

Mix the cornflour to a smooth paste with the sugar and 30ml/2 tablespoons of the milk. Bring the rest of the milk to the boil and add to the cornflour mixture. Mix until smooth, add the vanilla essence, return to the pan, stirring continuously until boiling, and simmer for one minute. Serve hot or cold.
Fat: Nil
Oil: Nil

Vanilla and Yoghurt Sauce

Equal quantities of cold vanilla sauce and home-made yoghurt can be whisked together to make a delightfully fresh-tasting sauce which goes well with cold cooked fruit or other cold puddings. Many people may prefer this recipe to cream substitutes.
Fat: Nil
Oil: Nil

Breakfasts

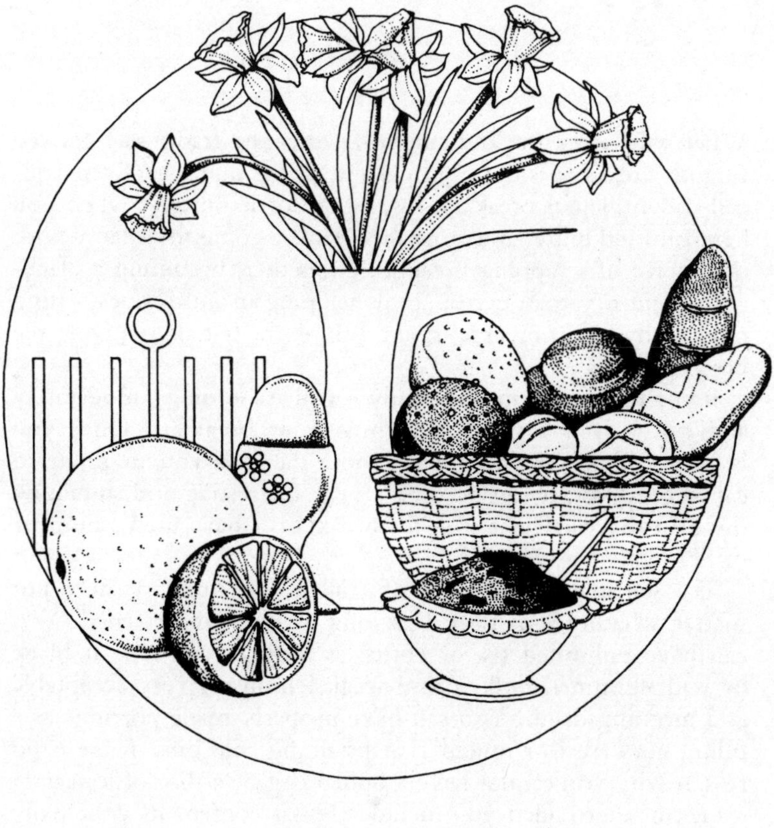

When you are on a low-animal-fat diet the traditional cooked English breakfast is quite simply out of the question. Even a so-called continental breakfast loses some of its interest when you have omitted butter and croissants. You're going to be faced with the choice of scrapping breakfast altogether, becoming a black-coffee-and-dry-toast person, or developing an entirely new eating philosophy about breakfasts; and I think the last alternative is the best.

If you tire easily, and especially if you are leading a moderately active life, it is a mistake to miss your breakfast. Once you begin to think quite differently about the food you are going to eat at breakfast, it can become a very interesting and sustaining meal. In my particular plan for breakfasts I have used a number of Scandinavian ideas.

Try starting with a glass of chilled fruit juice. It does not matter whether it is tinned as long as it is unsweetened. You can have unlimited tea or coffee as long as you take it black or with skimmed milk. I find weak lemon tea very acceptable as a morning drink. You can have properly made porridge as a filling hot cereal or muesli as a sustaining cold one. There is no reason why you cannot have a boiled egg or a slice of lean ham sometimes, provided you include the fat content in your daily allowance. Home-made yoghurt is another delicious and fat-free addition to breakfast, and the meal can be rounded off with a mouth-watering selection of home-made breads, oatcakes, bought crispbreads, marmalade, honey and home-made jellies.

Porridge

I find the mystique of making traditional Scottish porridge as fascinating as that of wine tasting. Successful porridge requires good judgement, a certain amount of time spent each morning and a considerable amount of manual dexterity. For each good portion of porridge you require 250ml/one breakfast cup of water and 60ml/a quarter of the same sized cup of medium oatmeal. Porridge oats are not an acceptable substitute for those who have eaten 'real' porridge. About 1ml/$\frac{1}{4}$ teaspoon of salt is needed for each portion of porridge, and an attempt should be made to convert the unconverted to eating porridge without sugar – black treacle is a good alternative. Traditionally, very hot porridge is put into a cold bowl and a small bowl of cold milk or cream is served separately. Each spoonful of porridge is dipped into the milk or cream before being eaten. Until the 1940s remote crofters would have milk with porridge during the winter until the cow 'went dry' and would then have black treacle.

Put the required measure of water into a very thick-bottomed pan and bring it to the boil. This is the point at which manual dexterity is required. Have the necessary measure of oatmeal in a dry cup near your left hand. With your right hand take either a small long-handled silver spoon or a long wooden handle with no spoon. (This is called different names in different parts of Scotland, including 'spurtle' and 'theevil'.) The stick must be used in a clockwise direction, and when a vortex is formed the oatmeal must be tipped by the left hand in a fine, steady stream slowly and continuously into the middle of the vortex. The stirring must be done steadily and in this way no lumps will form. When all the oatmeal is added, simmer uncovered for ten minutes. Add the requisite amount of salt and simmer for another ten minutes, after which the porridge is ready to be served.

Oatcakes

If you want to have a ready supply of oatcakes, good-quality ones may be bought in tins or packets. If you have the time to make them they are tasty but tend to crumble on keeping and are best eaten fresh.

100g/4oz oatmeal
10ml/1 dessertspoon SFS oil
about 50ml/2 fl oz hot water
1ml/¼ teaspoon salt
3ml/½ teaspoon baking powder
extra oatmeal for kneading and rolling

Mix all the ingredients together until a thick paste is formed. Turn this out on to a board and knead with oatmeal until it is of a suitable consistency for rolling. Roll out as thinly as possible and either cut into rounds about 70mm/2½in in diameter or cut round a saucer and score each large circle to be broken into four pieces after cooking. Heat a heavy iron griddle (girdle) on a low heat and cook the oatcakes for five minutes each side approximately or until dry. Leave to cool on a wire tray and eat while fresh with PUF margarine or low-fat cottage cheese.
Fat: Nil
Oil: 10g/2 teaspoons

Home-Made Muesli

500g/1lb porridge oats
25g/1oz oat flakes
75g/3oz sultanas
75g/3oz dried skimmed milk
50g/2oz ground nuts
50g/2oz wheat flakes
25g/1oz bran
75g/3oz raisins
50g/2oz demerara sugar

Mix all the ingredients together and store in an airtight container.
Fat: 20g/4 teaspoons
Oil: 5g/1 teaspoon

Wholemeal Bread

750g/1½lb stone-ground wholemeal flour
30g/1½oz dried yeast
15ml/3 teaspoons salt
about 900ml/1½ pints warm water
750g/1½lb strong white flour
15ml/1 tablespoon SFS oil
15ml/1 tablespoon molasses sugar

Mix together half the warm water, the dried yeast and the molasses sugar and leave to stand for about ten minutes until it is frothy. Put the flour and salt into a large bowl and make a well in the centre. Pour in the yeast mixture, the oil and the rest of the warm water and knead with a dough hook or by hand until an elastic dough is formed, adding more warm water if necessary. Cover the dough with a damp cloth and leave it in a warm place until it has doubled in size. Knead again, shape into loaves and put into two large greased bread tins. Leave the dough, again covered with a damp cloth, until it has doubled in size. Bake in an oven at 220°C/425°F/gas mark 7 for twenty-five minutes. Turn the oven down to 190°C/375°F/gas mark 5 and bake for another twenty minutes or until the loaf is well risen, golden brown in colour and sounds hollow if taken out of the tin and knocked with a knuckle on the under side.
Fat: Nil
Oil: 20g/4 teaspoons

Buckwheat Bread

We are fortunate enough to have a coarse buckwheat flour sent from a friend in the United States; but a similar flour may be bought from health food or real food stores in the United Kingdom. This recipe makes a delightfully light spongy bread but one which dries out in a short time, and one or two loaves are better frozen if not eaten quickly.

300g/10oz buckwheat flour
5ml/1 teaspoon salt
30g/1½oz dried yeast
10ml/2 teaspoons molasses
300g/10oz wholemeal flour
125g/5oz plain white flour
350ml/12 fl oz warm water
45ml/3 tablespoons SFS oil

Mix the dried yeast and the molasses until the mixture is smooth. Add the warm water. Mix all the dry ingredients together and add the yeast mixture and the oil. Knead by hand or mix with a dough hook until the mixture makes a smooth dough. Cover the dough with a damp towel and leave it in a warm place until it has doubled its size. Grease three oblong bread tins and divide the dough equally between them. Push the dough down with your knuckles to make an even surface and trim with whole buckwheat if it is available. Cover the tins with a damp cloth and leave again in a warm place until the dough has doubled in size. Bake the bread for thirty minutes in an oven at 200°C/400°F/gas mark 6.
Fat: Nil
Oil: 60g/12 teaspoons

Black Bread

This black bread is more like a richly flavoured malt bread than a continental rye. It may be difficult to get the dark rye flour advised, but it is delicious with lighter rye flour obtainable at most health food stores. Do not make the dough too moist or the bread will be too sticky.

500g/1lb dark or light rye flour
25g/1oz dried yeast
5ml/1 teaspoon salt
225g/8oz granary flour
600ml/1 pint warm skimmed milk
15ml/1 tablespoon molasses

Mix the dried yeast and molasses together until smooth and add the warm milk. Leave the mixture to stand until frothy. Put all the dry ingredients together and add the yeast mixture. Knead by hand or with a dough hook until a smooth dough is formed. Put it into a bowl, cover with a damp cloth and leave to stand in a warm place until the dough has doubled its size. Remove the dough from the bowl and knead again. Divide into two and form each part into a long loaf pointed at both ends. Put the two loaves on a large oiled baking sheet and leave again in a warm place until they have doubled in size. Bake in an oven at

200°C/400°F/gas mark 6 for about forty-five minutes. This bread keeps very well in a tightly sealed tin for over a week.
Fat: Nil
Oil: Nil

Granary Bread

750g/1½lb granary flour
5ml/1 teaspoon salt
7ml/½ tablespoon molasses sugar
20g/¾oz dried yeast
10ml/2 teaspoons SFS oil
350ml/12fl oz warm water

Put the dried yeast, molasses sugar and half the warm water in a bowl and leave for about ten minutes until the mixture is frothy. Put the flour, salt and oil in a mixing bowl and make a well in the centre. Pour in the yeast mixture and the rest of the water. Knead with a dough hook or by hand until a firm elastic dough is formed. Cover the dough with a damp cloth and leave in a warm place until it has doubled in size. Knead again and form into two round loaves. Put them on a greased baking sheet and return them to a warm place for a further thirty minutes. Bake them in an oven at 200°C/400°F/gas mark 6 for about thirty-five minutes.
Fat: Nil
Oil: 10g/2 teaspoons

Date and Walnut Bread

350g/12oz wholemeal flour
100g/4oz chopped dates
1 egg
90ml/6 tablespoons skimmed milk
100g/4oz soft dark brown sugar
100g/4oz chopped walnuts
60ml/4 tablespoons black treacle

Put the flour, sugar, dates and nuts together in a bowl. Beat the egg and add to the dry ingedients with the treacle and milk. Mix until of an even consistency and put into a large greased

bread tin. Bake at 160°C/325°F/gas mark 3 for about one and a half hours.
Fat: 15g/3 teaspoons
Oil: 40g/8 teaspoons

I am not able to leave the subject of breakfast without giving the recipes for three of our favourite jellies which are yours for the finding and the work. The nicest, I think, is elderberry and apple jelly; I once gave a precious pound jar of it to a charity bring-and-buy stall. As I walked away I heard one helper say to the other in that most English of English accents, 'She *says* you can eat it.'!

Elderberry and Apple Jelly

2·25l/2 quarts by volume of elderberries, removed from their stalks
water
1·5kg/3lb cooking apples
sugar
1 orange
1 stick cinnamon

The elderberries can be removed fairly rapidly from their stalks by pulling a fork through each cluster. Cut the apples into even-sized pieces, removing bruised or bad parts but not the cores. Put the fruit into a large pan and cover with water. Bring to the boil and simmer until the fruit can be reduced to a pulp with a potato masher. Put the fruit into a jelly bag and leave it to drain over night. Add 0·5kg/1lb granulated sugar to each pint of juice, warm in a pan over a low heat and stir until all the sugar is melted. Peel the orange and tie the peel and the cinnamon stick together and put in with the fruit and sugar. Add the juice of the orange, bring to the boil and boil rapidly until the jelly will set when tested – about twenty-five minutes. Remove the cinnamon and orange rind and pot while hot.
Fat: Nil
Oil: Nil

Quince Jelly

Unfortunately quinces are becoming a very rare fruit but a quince bush will grow and bear fruit very successfully in most parts of England if planted in a warm sunny corner of the garden.

2kg/4lb quinces
water
2 lemons
2·5kg/5lb cooking apples
sugar

Cut the fruit into even-sized pieces, discarding parts that are bruised or bad but not the cores. Cover with water, simmer, mush and drain as described in the elderberry and apple jelly recipe opposite. Add 0·5kg/1lb of granulated sugar to each 600ml/1 pint of juice and allow the mixture to warm gently, stirring until all the sugar is dissolved. Add the juice of the two lemons and the pared rind tied together with fine string. Boil until of a setting consistency and remove the rind before putting into pots.
Fat: Nil
Oil: Nil

Crab Apple Jelly

Unfortunately, with the wholesale destruction of our hedgerows, crab apples have become a rarity. The garden variety will make good jelly, often with a particularly pleasing colour.

crab apples
water
sugar

The method is the same as described for quince and no additions are required. The juice and sugar usually need to boil for about fifteen minutes before reaching the point of setting.
Fat: Nil
Oil: Nil

Soups

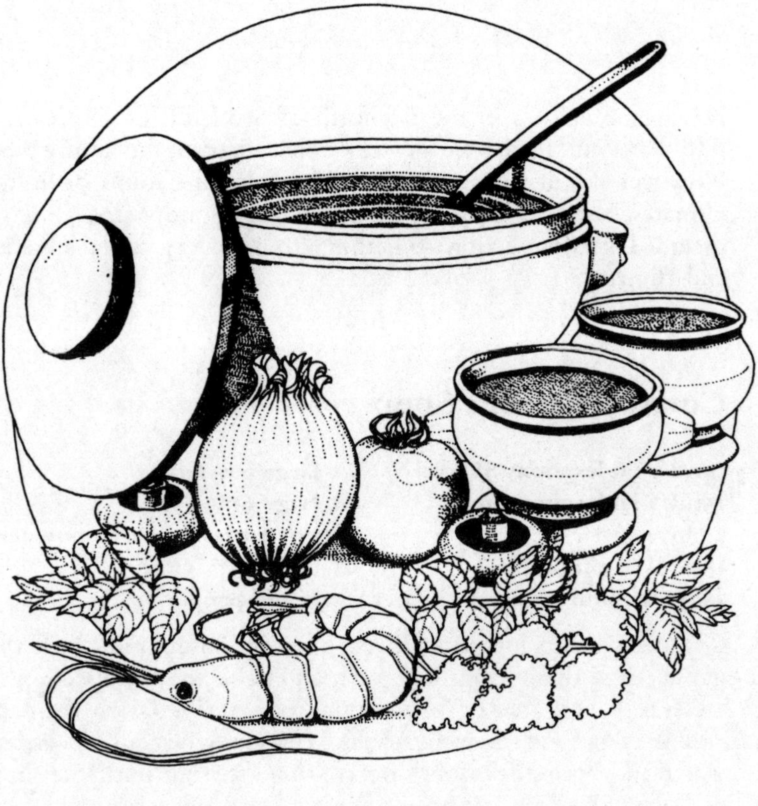

Having now lived in the far north of Scotland for six years, I find that soups have become very much a part of the family diet. However, I still harbour a great liking for the soups of hotter climates, such as gazpacho andaluz, and I hope that I have included in this section something to fit every taste, appetite and climate.

Curried Parsnip Soup

30ml/2 tablespoons SFS oil
15ml/1 tablespoon flour
1 clove garlic
1500ml/2½ pints water
25g/1oz skimmed milk powder
1 large parsnip
1 large onion
5ml/1 teaspoon curry powder
1 beef-stock cube
salt and pepper

Cut the parsnip into thin slices, dice the onion and crush the garlic. Heat the oil in a large pan and cook the chopped vegetables in it very gently for ten minutes with the lid on the pan. Add the flour and stir well. Add the curry powder, milk powder, water and beef-stock cube and continue stirring until the soup boils and thickens. Simmer the soup until the parsnip is very tender, which may be forty minutes. Put the soup through an electric blender, add the salt and pepper to taste and reheat before serving.

Fat: Nil
Oil: 40g/8 teaspoons

Gazpacho Andaluz

50g/2oz fresh brown breadcrumbs
2 cloves garlic
900ml/1½ pints tinned tomato juice
salt and pepper
croutons fried in SFS oil
45ml/3 tablespoons red wine vinegar
1 green pepper
1 cucumber
300ml/½ pint chilled water
60ml/4 tablespoons SFS oil
1 onion

Soak the freshly prepared breadcrumbs in the vinegar. Peel the cucumber and cut half of it into cubes and put into an electric blender. Chop the garlic, onion and green pepper and add to the cucumber. Add the soaked breadcrumbs and blend until the mixture is of a smooth consistency. Add the oil drop by drop, keeping the blender working. Add the salt and pepper and put the blended mixture into a serving dish. Add the tomato juice and water and check the seasoning and the amount of vinegar. Chill the soup well in the refrigerator. Dice the rest of the cucumber and the other half of the green pepper. Put these and the croutons in separate bowls and serve with the soup.
Fat: Nil
Oil: 80g/16 teaspoons

Brown Onion Soup

Traditionally this delicious soup should be served with Parmesan cheese, but unfortunately this cheese is very high in animal fat. The choice is to serve grated Parmesan – fresh, of course – in *small* quantities; or depart from tradition and try the Italian Mozzarella cheese which is lower in fat and which we find an acceptable alternative.

3 large onions
30ml/2 tablespoons flour
150ml/¼ pint dry white wine
croutons fried in SFS oil
30ml/2 tablespoons SFS oil
900ml/1½ pints water
salt and pepper
Mozzarella cheese

Slice the onions thinly. Put the oil in a large thick-bottomed

pan and add the onions. Cook slowly, turning frequently, until the onions are a pleasant golden brown – this needs some patience because they need adequate cooking to create the right flavour and colour but overcooking makes the soup bitter. Add the flour and cook for another five minutes. Boil the wine and water together and add to the onion mixture. Stir until the soup comes back to the boil, season and then simmer gently for twenty minutes. Just before serving, float the Mozzarella on the top. Serve the croutons separately.
Fat: Nil
Oil: 40g/8 teaspoons

Lentil Soup

Traditionally a Scottish soup, I find this tastier made with brown lentils. They need no soaking and salt should not be added until the lentils have softened. A stock can be made with a ham bone, or a cube of ham bouillon may be used which is sometimes more practical.

150g/6oz lentils
1 large potato
salt and pepper to taste
1500ml/2½ pints water or ham stock
1 ham bouillon cube (if using water)
1 large carrot
1 medium onion
75g/3oz dried skimmed milk

Dice the onion, potato and carrot and put them with the lentils and the stock or water into a thick-bottomed pan. Add the bouillon cube if being used. Bring to the boil slowly and simmer gently for about two hours. Put all the ingredients, including the dried milk, through a blender until the soup is of the desired consistency. Return to the pan, adjust the seasoning; this soup often needs no extra salt. Serve very hot with croutons cooked in sunflower seed oil if desired.
Fat: Nil
Oil: Nil

Mushroom Soup

This soup is tastiest when made with field mushrooms. If these are not obtainable, mushrooms may be grown at home from one of the prepared kits with very little trouble. These mushrooms can be eaten as soon as picked and make tastier dishes than commercially grown mushrooms.

1 onion
225g/8oz mushrooms
450ml/¾ pint prepared skimmed milk
½ chicken stock cube
chopped fresh parsley to garnish
30ml/2 tablespoons SFS oil
35g/1½oz flour
450ml/¾ pint water
salt and pepper

Chop the onion very finely and cook gently in the oil until it is transparent but not coloured. Add the chopped mushrooms and cook for a further four minutes. Stir in the flour, cooking for another minute. Add the milk, water, stock cube and seasoning. Stir continuously until the soup boils and thickens. Turn down the heat and simmer for ten minutes. Garnish with the chopped parsley before serving.
Fat: Nil
Oil: 40g/8 teaspoons

Cullen Skink

225g/8oz smoked haddock
500g/1lb mashed potato
1 onion
600ml/1 pint skimmed milk
salt and pepper

Poach the haddock with the finely chopped onion in a pan with enough water to cover the fish. About ten minutes is usually enough time for the fish to begin to flake away from the bones. Remove the fish, flake the flesh and put the bones back in the pan to cook for about an hour. Add the fish and milk to the fish stock. Add enough mashed potato to make the soup of a thick-cream consistency and season to taste.
Fat: 5g/1 teaspoon
Oil: Nil

Prawn and Sweetcorn Chowder

15ml/1 tablespoon SFS oil
25g/1oz lean ham
100g/4oz frozen prawns
½ chicken stock cube
15ml/1 tablespoon arrowroot
2 small onions
225g/8oz frozen sweetcorn kernels
600ml/1 pint water
300ml/½ pint skimmed milk
salt and pepper

Chop the onions very finely and soften them in the oil but do not allow them to brown. Cut the ham into small pieces and add it to the onions with the sweetcorn, water, chicken stock cube and seasoning. Cook gently until the corn is tender – about twenty minutes. Add the thawed prawns and simmer for another five minutes. Mix the arrowroot to a thin paste with some of the milk and then add to the hot mixture with the rest of the milk and bring back to the boil. Boil very gently for a further two minutes before serving.
Fat: 10g/2 teaspoons
Oil: 20g/4 teaspoons

Italian Vegetable Soup

50g/2oz dried haricot beans
1 stick of celery
1 carrot
2 tomatoes
7ml/½ tablespoon tomato puree
1 chicken stock cube
50g/2oz spaghetti
salt and pepper
1 onion
2 courgettes
100g/4oz French beans
1 potato
30ml/2 tablespoons SFS oil
1500ml/2½ pints water
2 cloves garlic
5ml/1 teaspoon basil
chopped fresh parsley to garnish

Soak the dried haricot beans in water without salt for twenty-four hours. Simmer them in fresh water for about one and a half hours and drain them. Heat the oil in a large pan. Dice the onion, celery, carrot, courgettes and tomatoes. Crush the garlic and cut the French beans into short lengths. Add all these vegetables to the hot oil and cook gently for ten minutes. Stir

them frequently and do not allow them to brown. Add the water, crumbled stock cube, tomato puree, basil and seasoning. Simmer the soup for about thirty-five minutes. Dice the potato and break the spaghetti into short lengths, add to the soup and cook for another fifteen minutes. Add the cooked and drained haricot beans and reheat before serving, garnished with chopped fresh parsley.
Fat: Nil
Oil: 40g/8 teaspoons

Yoghurt Soup

1 large cucumber
3ml/½ teaspoon paprika
salt and pepper
300g/10oz home-made yoghurt
1 clove garlic

Peel the cucumber and cut it into pieces. Put all the ingredients into an electric blender and blend until smooth. Chill well before serving. Chopped chives make a good garnish if available.
Fat: Nil
Oil: Nil

Mushroom and Potato Soup

2 onions
75g/3oz mushrooms
900ml/1½ pints skimmed milk
15ml/1 tablespoon arrowroot
30ml/2 tablespoons SFS oil
1kg/2lb potatoes
1 bay leaf
30ml/2 tablespoons skimmed milk
salt and pepper

Heat the oil in a large pan. Dice the onions and potatoes and cook gently in the oil for about twenty minutes, but do not let them brown. Add the 900ml/1½ pints milk and bay leaf and simmer very gently for about thirty minutes. When the vegetables are well cooked, remove the bay leaf and put the soup through an electric blender until it is quite smooth. Chop the mushrooms in thin slices and add them to the soup. Mix the arrowroot to a

paste with the 30ml/2 tablespoons milk, pour a small amount of the boiling soup on to it, return the mixture to the pan and bring to the boil stirring continuously. Simmer for five minutes. Season to taste.
Fat: Nil
Oil: 40g/8 teaspoons

Vegetable and Prawn Soup

1 onion
75g/3oz frozen peas
30ml/2 tablespoons SFS oil
1 clove garlic
soy sauce
1 carrot
1 medium-sized courgette
1200ml/2 pints water
salt and pepper
100g/4oz frozen prawns

Dice all the vegetables and crush the clove of garlic. Heat the oil and cook the diced vegetables, garlic and peas gently in the oil for ten minutes, stirring them and not allowing them to brown. Add the water and simmer for thirty minutes. Put the soup through an electric blender until of the desired consistency. Add the salt and pepper, the thawed prawns, and soy sauce to taste. Bring to the boil and simmer for another five minutes before serving.
Fat: 2·5g/½ teaspoon
Oil: 40g/8 teaspoons

Partan Bree

If you have a supply of crabs and do not mind cooking and dressing them yourself, this soup is better made with fresh crab; otherwise a tin of crab will do adequately. I am happy to cook crabs if they arrive at my back door but am not too keen on driving home from the harbour with five large crustacea rampaging on the floor of the car under my seat, waving their murderous claws alongside the gear lever.

flesh from 1 fresh crab or 1 225g/8oz tin crab
600ml/1 pint water
10ml/2 teaspoons anchovy essence
good pinch pepper
75g/3oz rice
600ml/1 pint skimmed milk
25g/1oz dried skimmed milk

Boil the rice in the milk until it is well cooked. Add the crab meat and put the mixture through the electric blender until it is smooth. Add the water and anchovy essence. Taste and season. If you want the soup of a creamier consistency whisk in 25g/1oz dried skimmed milk.
Fat: 5g/1 teaspoon
Oil: Nil

Borsch with Sour Cream

1 onion
150g/6oz finely shredded cabbage
30ml/2 tablespoons tomato puree
15ml/1 tablespoon sugar
1 ham bouillon cube
1200ml/2 pints water
1 carrot
1 large beetroot
15ml/1 tablespoon red wine vinegar
15ml/1 tablespoon SFS oil
salt and pepper
sour-cream substitute (see p.23)

Dice the onion and carrot. Peel the beetroot and slice into long thin matchstick-shaped pieces. Heat the oil in a large pan and fry the vegetables for ten minutes. Add the rest of the ingredients, apart from the sour-cream substitute, and simmer for thirty minutes. Put in the electric blender for a few seconds but do not blend until the consistency is uniform. Reheat and serve with a spoonful of sour-cream substitute on each helping.
Fat: Nil
Oil: 20g/4 teaspoons

Cream of Sweetcorn and Tuna

My family has a preference for soups with interesting things in them and this one fills the bill very well. The dry sherry is optional.

15ml/1 tablespoon SFS oil
½ chicken stock cube
100g/4oz tinned or frozen sweetcorn
15ml/1 tablespoon dry sherry
15ml/1 tablespoon flour
450ml/¾ pint skimmed milk
100g/4oz tuna
salt and pepper

Melt the oil in a pan and stir in the flour. Add the milk and stock cube and bring to the boil, stirring all the time. Boil for two minutes. Add the sweetcorn. Take the tuna out of the tin and drain away all the oil. Flake the fish finely and add it to the soup. Add the sherry and season to taste. Reheat, but do not boil it again.
Fat: 20g/4 teaspoons
Oil: 20g/4 teaspoons

Jerusalem Artichoke Soup

1kg/2lb Jerusalem artichokes
30ml/2 tablespoons SFS oil
600ml/1 pint water
45ml/3 tablespoons cold skimmed milk
2 onions
450ml/¾ pint skimmed milk
15ml/1 tablespoon cornflour
salt and pepper

Peel the artichokes and cut them into even-sized pieces. Cut up the onions finely and add both vegetables to the heated oil. Simmer the vegetables in the fat for fifteen minutes, but do not allow them to brown. Add the water, season to taste, cover and simmer for thirty minutes. Put the mixture into an electric blender and mix until the consistency of a fine puree. Put the mixture back into the pan and add the 450ml/¾ pint milk. Bring to the boil. Mix the cornflour to a thin paste with the 45ml/3 tablespoons of cold milk and pour on some of the boiling mixture. Return to the pan, bring back to the boil and simmer for a further five minutes, stirring continuously before serving.
Fat: Nil
Oil: 40g/8 teaspoons

Pea and Ham Soup

I should have liked to include a recipe for Swedish Thursday soup which I first tasted on a Finnish cargo boat. Unfortunately in its original form it is too rich in fat for inclusion in this book and I am using a much modified version.

350g/12oz split peas
2 leeks
1 carrot
salt and pepper
50g/2oz lean ham
30ml/2 tablespoons SFS oil
1 onion

Soak the split peas in plenty of cold water overnight. Drain them, cover them with fresh cold water and bring them to the boil slowly. Dice the onion and carrot and cut the leeks into thin slices. Add the vegetables to the cooking peas and continue to simmer until the peas are tender. Put the soup in an electric blender, but blend only for a few seconds. Add the diced ham, adjust the seasoning and reheat.
Fat: Nil
Oil: 40g/8 teaspoons

Carrot and Orange Soup

15ml/1 tablespoon PUF margarine
2 onions
1 chicken bouillon cube
juice of $\frac{1}{2}$ an orange
6 carrots
900ml/1$\frac{1}{2}$ pints water
50g/2oz skimmed milk powder
salt and pepper

Dice the carrots and onions. Heat the margarine and cook the vegetables very gently in the fat until they are soft but not browned. Add the water and stock cube and simmer for an hour. Put the mixture in an electric blender and mix until very smooth. Add the milk powder and continue blending. Return the soup to the saucepan on the stove and reheat. Season to taste. Add the orange juice immediately before serving.
Fat: 5g/1 teaspoon
Oil: Nil

Cream of Celery Soup

1 head celery
45ml/3 tablespoons SFS oil
8 peppercorns
900ml/1½ pints skimmed milk
30ml/2 tablespoons cornflour
1 onion
2 bay leaves
2 blades mace
45ml/3 tablespoons cold skimmed milk

Cut the celery and onion into small pieces and cook them gently in the warmed oil for about thirty minutes until they are quite tender. Heat the 900ml/1½ pints milk with the peppercorns, bay leaves and mace for about twenty minutes at nearly boiling point. Push the softened vegetables through a fine sieve; an electric blender is unsuitable. Strain the heated milk. Mix the cornflour to a smooth paste with the 45ml/3 tablespoons cold milk. Pour on the hot strained milk and add the sieved vegetables. Bring to the boil, stirring continuously and allow to simmer for two minutes before serving.
Fat: Nil
Oil: 60g/12 teaspoons

Cream of Asparagus Soup

Of course, this should be made with fresh asparagus, but if you find it impossible, as we do, to get fresh asparagus, a quite acceptable version can be made with a large tin of this vegetable.

1 bundle fresh asparagus or **1 large (500g/16oz) tin asparagus**
900ml/1½ pints skimmed milk
45ml/3 tablespoons cold skimmed milk
1 small onion
40g/2 tablespoons cornflour
salt and pepper

Cut the asparagus and onion into small pieces and simmer in the milk until the vegetables are tender. This will take about thirty minutes. Mix the cornflour and the 45ml/3 tablespoons of cold milk to a smooth paste. Pass the vegetable mixture through a blender and add some of it to the paste. Return the whole to the saucepan,

bring back to the boil, stirring continuously, season and simmer for two minutes.
Fat: Nil
Oil: Nil

Mussel Broth

1 quart (about 60) mussels
5ml/1 teaspoon mixed herbs
900ml/1$\frac{1}{2}$ pints water
30ml/2 tablespoons SFS oil
15ml/1 tablespoon lemon juice
1 clove garlic
1 glass dry white wine
salt and pepper
225g/8oz tomatoes or 1 small (225g/8oz) tin tomatoes
30ml/2 tablespoons cornflour
50g/2oz diced mixed vegetables
chopped fresh parsley to garnish

Leave the mussels in a large bowl of cold water overnight and in the morning scrub them vigorously with a brush to remove the whiskery pieces on them, discarding any which are not tightly closed. Put the mussels into a large pan with the wine, mixed herbs and lemon juice. Cover and bring to the boil, turning the shellfish frequently. When the mussels are all opened, remove any remaining beard from them and strain the liquid through muslin and set it aside. Put the oil and diced vegetables into a clean pan and cook gently until the vegetables are soft. Add the cornflour and stir well. Put the tomatoes through an electric blender and add them to the vegetable mixture with the water, seasoning, crushed clove of garlic and stock from the mussels. Bring to the boil and simmer for five minutes. Remove the mussels from their shells and add them to the mixture. Heat the broth but do not boil again as this tends to make the mussels rubbery. Garnish with parsley.
Fat: 5g/1 teaspoon
Oil: 40g/8 teaspoons

Smoked Trout Soup

I am indebted for the following recipe to an engineer friend who prefers to remain anonymous. He started his life-long interest in gourmet cooking while at a boy's boarding school where he managed to build a secret kitchen in the attic above his dormitory. I have had to adapt one or two of the original ingredients but hope that I have made up for the changes by quotations from his highly individual description of this wonderful soup.

1 wine glass whisky
1 onion
50g/2oz brown breadcrumbs
1 bay leaf
5ml/1 teaspoon sugar
25g/1oz dried skimmed milk
2 smoked trout
1 carrot
15ml/1 tablespoon tomato puree
5ml/1 teaspoon salt
2ml/½ teaspoon fennel seeds, crushed
1200ml/2 pints water

Put the glass of whisky, water, trout, salt and bay leaf into a large pan. Cover, bring to the boil slowly and simmer for twenty minutes. Remove the fish from the liquid. Chop the onion finely, grate the carrot and add these to the liquid with the breadcrumbs, crushed fennel seeds and tomato puree. Simmer for a further twenty minutes. Meanwhile, remove the skin from the fish (and give to dog), separate the flesh, taking care to remove the bones, and mince the flesh finely. Remove the pan from the heat and add the minced fish. Remove the bay leaf and liquidise the soup with the dried milk powder, thinning with a little water if necessary. Adjust the seasoning before serving.
Fat: 10g/2 teaspoons
Oil: Nil

Other Starters

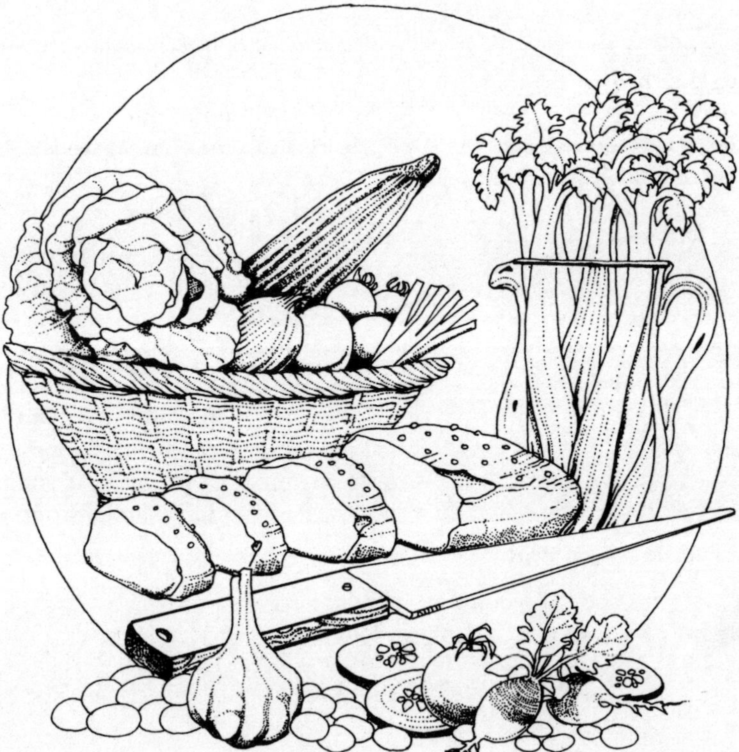

Perhaps I should have begun with starters and put soups in second place, because in our family they definitely do take second place. Other starters can include such a wide range of dishes, and so many can be made without any animal fat. I am assuming that the following recipes, whether hot or cold, will be used for the introduction to a main meal, but many of them may be used equally well for a light lunch or supper.

I have included one or two recipes which have a certain amount of animal fat, such as those containing herring, but in our family these are considered so outstandingly good that it is thought worth eating them and cutting down on other animal fat for that day.

A collection of these recipes, served with an assortment of salads, makes a mouth-watering informal menu for a buffet supper or lunch.

Salad Niçoise

Unfortunately some of the classic ingredients of this delicious salad are comparatively high in fat; however, we still enjoy eating it with reduced quantities of the restricted foods and some members of the family can cheat.

heart of 1 lettuce
1 heart chicory
½ cucumber
2 hard-boiled eggs
1 green pepper
French dressing (see p.22) with 1 clove garlic crushed in it
1 heart celery
4 tomatoes
black olives, or green if black are not obtainable
4 tinned anchovy fillets
100g/4oz tinned tuna fish

Break the lettuce heart into pieces. Cut the chicory and celery into chunks and divide each tomato into four. Quarter each hard-boiled egg. Strain the oil from the tuna fish and break the fish into largish pieces. Halve the anchovy fillets. Take the seeds out of the pepper and slice it finely. Cut the cucumber into chunks. Put all the ingredients together. Dress immediately before eating.

Fat: 20g/4 teaspoons
Oil: 40g/8 teaspoons

Baked Courgettes and Tomatoes

2 medium-sized courgettes
225g/8oz low-fat cottage cheese
5ml/1 teaspoon basil
15ml/1 tablespoon grated Parmesan cheese
1 small onion
7ml/½ tablespoon concentrated tomato puree
salt and pepper
15ml/1 tablespoon SFS oil

Heat the oil and cook the sliced courgettes and diced onion very slowly until the onions are soft and transparent. Put the cottage cheese in an electric blender and blend until quite smooth. Add the tomato puree, basil and seasoning. Put the vegetables in the base of an oven-to-table casserole and spread the cottage-cheese mixture over them. Sprinkle the Parmesan cheese over the top and bake in an oven at 180°C/350°F/gas mark 4 for thirty minutes.
Fat: 5g/1 teaspoon
Oil: 20g/4 teaspoons

Cod's Roe Pâté

Cod's roe has become something of a rarity; we can still buy it occasionally but this dish may be made with tinned roe if fresh is not obtainable.

150g/6oz fresh or tinned cod's roe
15ml/1 tablespoon SFS oil
1 clove garlic
25g/1oz fresh brown breadcrumbs
15ml/1 tablespoon lemon juice
30ml/2 tablespoons home-made substitute mayonnaise (see p.24)
salt and pepper

Enclose the cod's roe in a piece of muslin and cook it in boiling salted water for twenty minutes. Take it out of the water and allow it to drain until cold. Remove the skin and put the roe in an electric blender. Add the oil a little at a time, with the blender running. Crush the clove of garlic, add this with the seasoning, lemon juice, breadcrumbs and mayonnaise, and continue to blend for about two minutes until the mixture is very smooth. Leave

it in a serving bowl in the refrigerator overnight. Serve the pâté with thin slices of brown toast or home-made bread.
Fat: 10g/2 teaspoons
Oil: 20g/4 teaspoons

Hot Baked Grapefruit

2 grapefruit
40ml/4 dessertspoons demerara sugar
40ml/4 dessertspoons dry sherry
4 small dabs PUF margarine

Cut the grapefruit in half. Remove the central core and cut the flesh away from the pith with a sharp knife. Cut the flesh into bite-sized portions. Add the sherry and demerara sugar and put one dab of margarine in the centre of each grapefruit. Put each grapefruit in a small oven-to-table bowl and put about 8cm/3in under a hot grill. This will allow the grapefruit time to cook through before the top begins to caramelise. Serve hot.
Fat: Negligible
Oil: Nil

Smoked Haddock Soufflé

A fairly substantial first course to a meal and one which is also useful for a light supper.

225g/8oz smoked haddock fillets
1 onion
15ml/1 tablespoon cornflour
1 egg
45 ml/3 tablespoons cold skimmed milk
15ml/1 tablespoon SFS oil
a variable amount of dried skimmed milk to poach
pepper
100g/4oz low-fat cottage cheese

Poach the smoked haddock fillets in enough made-up dried milk to cover them. When the flesh is coming away from the skin, remove the fish from the liquid, skin and remove any bones. Flake

the fish into fairly small pieces. Chop the onion finely and soften it without browning in the hot oil. When the onion is soft, make up the milk in which the fish has been cooked to 300ml/½ pint and add it to the onions. Bring the mixture to the boil, stirring continuously, and simmer for two minutes. Blend the cornflour with the 45ml/3 tablespoons of cold skimmed milk and pour the boiling mixture on to it, stirring well. Put the cottage cheese in an electric blender and blend until quite smooth. Separate the egg. Beat the yolk into the milk mixture and add the cheese and fish. Beat the white of the egg and fold it into the fish mixture. Add pepper to taste. Bake in an oven at 180°C/350°F/gas mark 4 for thirty minutes, when it should be risen and a golden brown. Serve immediately.
Fat: 10g/2 teaspoons
Oil: 20g/4 teaspoons

Salt Herring in Sour Cream

Herring are relatively high in animal fat but you do not need to eat much as a starter and this recipe is particularly delicious.

4 salt herring
30ml/2 tablespoons red wine vinegar
5ml/1 teaspoon made English mustard
pepper
1 ripe apple
1 onion
30ml/2 tablespoons SFS oil
5ml/1 teaspoon sugar
50g/2oz sour-cream substitute

Soak the herring in cold water for at least twenty-four hours, changing the water several times. Remove the heads from the fish, gut them, skin them and cut one whole fillet from each side. With a sharp knife none of this is too difficult. Mix the oil, vinegar, sugar and seasonings and marinate the fillets of herring in this mixture for another twenty-four hours. Serve the fillets each garnished with a whirl of whipped sour-cream substitute and grated apple. This dish is particularly delicious if served with freshly home-baked rye bread.
Fat: 40g/8 teaspoons
Oil: 40g/8 teaspoons

Pickled Salt Herring

4 salt herring
100ml/4oz distilled vinegar
5ml/1 teaspoon allspice
2 onions
150ml/6oz water
125g/5oz granulated sugar

Soak the herring in cold water for at least twenty-four hours, changing the water several times. Remove the heads, guts and skins from the herring. Cut each fish across the body into pieces about 4cm/1½in long, put in a serving bowl; cut the onions into rings and arrange on the top. Make the pickling fluid by boiling the water, vinegar, sugar and allspice together for two minutes. Allow to cool and pour over the herring. Leave the pickled fish overnight in a refrigerator and serve them with home-made wholemeal bread.
Fat: 40g/8 teaspoons
Oil: Nil

Mushroom Soufflé

Delicious as a hot starter if you have the gift of getting your family to the table at the right moment; also excellent as a light supper dish. I prefer to make this with home-grown mushrooms, but it can be made with bought fresh ones or even with thawed frozen ones.

15ml/1 tablespoon SFS oil
¼ chicken stock cube
1 small onion
3 eggs
30ml/2 tablespoons flour
salt
dash Tabasco sauce
225g/8oz mushrooms
300ml/½ pint skimmed milk

Dice the onion finely and cook gently in the oil until transparent. Add the flour and stir until smooth. Add the warmed milk and stock cube and stir continuously until it has come to the boil and simmered for two minutes. Separate the egg yolks and whites. Beat the yolks into the sauce, one at a time. Add the finely sliced mushrooms and the seasoning. Whisk the egg whites until they are stiff and fold gently into the mushroom mixture. Bake in

an oven at 180°C/350°F/gas mark 4 for forty minutes until the soufflé is a golden brown and well risen. Serve immediately.
Fat: 15g/3 teaspoons
Oil: 20g/4 teaspoons

French-Style Tomato Salad

I have never eaten tomato salad in the United Kingdom which bears any resemblance to the glory of a real French tomato salad. Perhaps it is made from a different type of tomato and we have now heard that *the* tomato to use is one called Marmande so we are growing it. It is still too early to give a verdict on the product. For the moment I continue to buy tomatoes which are fairly large, not too ripe and of an even colour and consistency. I do not peel them. I cut them across the grain. The onions need to be strong-flavoured, the dressing well salted and the parsley fresh. The perfect tomato salad is the best starter I know for a meal.

1kg/2lb tomatoes
15ml/1 tablespoon red wine vinegar
5ml/1 teaspoon salt
225g/8oz onions
45ml/3 tablespoons SFS oil
5ml/1 teaspoon French mustard
chopped fresh parsley to garnish

Do not peel the tomatoes. Cut them into even-sized slices across the grain and arrange on individual plates. Cut the onion into fine rings and arrange on top of the tomatoes. Make the dressing by blending the oil, vinegar, mustard and salt. Pour over the salad and garnish with the chopped parsley before serving.
Fat: Nil
Oil: 60g/12 teaspoons

Liver Pâté

Liver pâté should have some fat bacon in it, but because of its fat content I have omitted this and put in ¼ ham bouillon cube to improve the flavour.

350g/12oz calf's liver
2 cloves garlic
$\frac{1}{4}$ ham bouillon cube
5ml/1 teaspoon anchovy essence

For the sauce

2 generous slices onion
15ml/1 tablespoon PUF margarine
1 bay leaf
6 peppercorns
300ml/$\frac{1}{2}$ pint skimmed milk
15ml/1 tablespoon flour
1 blade mace
salt and pepper

Put the peppercorns, mace, bay leaf and slices of onion in the milk and bring to near-boiling. Leave hot for about twenty minutes. Heat the margarine in another saucepan and stir in the flour. Strain the milk and add it to the fat and flour. Stir continuously and bring it to the boil. Boil for two minutes and season to taste. Put the liver and garlic through a mincer twice and add it to the sauce with the ham bouillon and anchovy essence. Mix well and put in a greased mould and cover with foil. Stand this in a tin of water and cook it in an oven at 150°C/300°F/gas mark 2 for forty-five minutes. Allow to cool and serve it with freshly made brown toast or home-made brown bread.
Fat: 12·5g/2$\frac{1}{2}$ teaspoons
Oil: 10g/2 teaspoons

Crudités

The most French and delicious of starters can be made with a great variety of grated raw vegetables served with a well-flavoured French dressing. I list some vegetables below, but you may find many more which are both available and delicious eaten raw.

1 raw beetroot
1 carrot
2 onions
a few radishes
1 red pepper
$\frac{1}{2}$ small red cabbage
2 small new turnips
$\frac{1}{2}$ cucumber
1 green pepper
15ml/1 tablespoon SFS oil

45ml/3 tablespoons red wine vinegar
5ml/1 teaspoon salt
5ml/1 teaspoon mustard
1 clove garlic

Grate the beetroot, cabbage, carrot and turnips. Slice the onions, peppers and cucumber thinly. Arrange attractively either on one large serving plate or on individual plates. Put the oil, wine vinegar, garlic, mustard and salt through an electric blender and pour over the vegetables.
Fat: Nil
Oil: 20g/4 teaspoons

Cottage Cheese and Fruit Salad

I first tasted this delicious mixture in the Erawan Hotel in Bangkok. It was served by elegantly dressed Thai girls in the exquisite garden in the centre of the hotel building, with the sound of the fountains in the background. Many of the fruits used there will not be available in the United Kingdom but others may be substituted at your discretion.

500g/1lb low-fat cottage cheese
2 fresh oranges *or* 1 small tin mandarins if liked
a few small white grapes
1 grapefruit
crisp lettuce leaves
2 bananas
225g/8oz strawberries

Peel the grapefruit and oranges. Cut them into slices across the grain of the sections and divide each slice into quarters, removing all stringy parts and pips. Peel and slice the bananas. Serve the salad on individual plates, putting a portion of cottage cheese and portions of the various fruits each on its own small lettuce leaf. This salad is not served with any dressing.
Fat: Nil
Oil: Nil

Red Bean Salad

An unusual first course and one which supplies a certain amount of protein in the beans.

100g/4oz dried red beans
½ green pepper
1 small onion
salt and pepper

For the dressing

30ml/2 tablespoons SFS oil
1 small onion, chopped
15ml/1 tablespoon chopped fresh parsley
7ml/½ tablespoon tarragon
5ml/1 teaspoon sugar
salt and pepper
30ml/2 tablespoons red wine vinegar
2 cloves garlic
7ml/½ tablespoon chopped basil
1ml/¼ teaspoon chilli powder
dash Tabasco sauce

Soak the red beans overnight. Put them in a pan with fresh water, the chopped green pepper and onion and simmer them until tender – about two hours. When they are cooked season them to taste. Pour off the water and allow the beans to cool.

Put the vinegar, seasoning, onion, garlic, sugar and chilli powder in an electric blender and blend them until smooth. Add the chopped herbs. Pour the dressing over the beans and mix well before serving.

Fat: Nil
Oil: 40g/8 teaspoons

Prawn Salad

My own family's passion for prawns, as well as cockles and mussels, started in the days when we spent all our free time on the north Norfolk coast. The sands at Brancaster and the prawn nets were a routine part of our life, along with sailing, and so was the eating of all the goodies.

100g/4oz fresh or frozen prawns
50g/2oz diced cucumber
50g/2oz diced cooked new or tinned potatoes
a few pieces of lettuce heart

30ml/2 tablespoons home-made mayonnaise
7ml/½ tablespoon concentrated tomato puree
a few black olives

Mix the prawns, potato and cucumber. Blend the mayonnaise with the tomato puree. Line attractive small serving dishes or ramekins with the lettuce heart. Mix the prawns, vegetables and sauce and spoon over the lettuce. Garnish with the black olives and chill before serving.
Fat: 2·5g/½ teaspoon
Oil: 10g/2 teaspoons

Cucumber and Cottage Cheese Mousse

A very light and refreshing starter for a heavy meal or a light meal for a hot day.

1 cucumber
15g/½oz gelatine
125g/5oz home-made yoghurt
½ small onion
chopped fresh chives to garnish
225g/8oz low-fat cottage cheese
45ml/3 tablespoons water
2 egg whites
salt and pepper

Peel the cucumber and dice it finely. Dissolve the gelatine in the water over a very low heat. Put the cottage cheese, yoghurt, salt and pepper and finely chopped onion in an electric blender and blend until smooth. Add the dissolved gelatine and mix well. Mix together the cucumber and cottage-cheese mixture, fold in the stiffly beaten egg whites and leave in the refrigerator for several hours to set. Garnish with chopped chives.
Fat: Nil
Oil: Nil

Prawn and Orange Cocktail

125g/5oz home-made yoghurt
1 orange
7ml/½ tablespoon chopped fresh parsley
5ml/1 teaspoon Worcester sauce
100g/4oz fresh or frozen prawns
2ml/½ teaspoon paprika
salt
a few lettuce leaves

The sauce for this can be made in advance and chilled but the prawns should not be added until shortly before serving. Mix together the yoghurt, Worcester sauce, seasonings and herbs. Peel the orange, cut into slices across the fruit and cut each slice into quarters. Put some small lettuce leaves in the bottom of each serving dish. Add the orange and the prawns to the sauce, spoon on to the lettuce base and serve.
Fat: 2·5g/½ teaspoon
Oil: Nil

Melon, Grapefruit and Tomato Salad

1 ripe melon
225g/8oz tomatoes
7ml/½ tablespoon caster sugar or to taste
2 grapefruit
2ml/½ teaspoon ground ginger

Peel the grapefruit so that no pith is left on the flesh. Cut it into slices across the direction of the segments and cut each slice into quarters, removing the central tough part and all the pips. Make sure you keep all the juice. Remove the flesh from the melon, discarding the seeds, and cut into bite-sized pieces. Remove the skin from the tomatoes, cut into quarters and take out the seeds. Put all the fruit together and sprinkle the caster sugar and ginger over the mixture. Leave in the refrigerator until well chilled and then serve in individual dishes.
Fat: Nil
Oil: Nil

Mushrooms in White Wine

This is a particularly favourite recipe with my family and large quantities tend to be eaten.

500g/1lb small button mushrooms
45ml/3 tablespoons SFS oil
salt and pepper
2ml/½ teaspoon ground coriander seeds
2 bay leaves
100g/4oz tomatoes
100ml/4 fl oz dry white wine
2ml/½ teaspoon thyme
1 clove garlic

Remove the skin from the tomatoes, cut them into quarters and discard the seeds. Wash the mushrooms. Put the wine, oil, seasoning, garlic and herbs in a pan, bring to the boil and simmer for five minutes. Add the mushrooms and cut-up tomatoes, cover the pan and cook very gently for a further five minutes. Remove the vegetables and put them in an attractive serving dish. Bring the remaining liquid to the boil and cook uncovered until it has halved its volume. Pour the mixture over the vegetables and serve when well chilled.
Fat: Nil
Oil: 60g/12 teaspoons

Salads and Vegetable Dishes

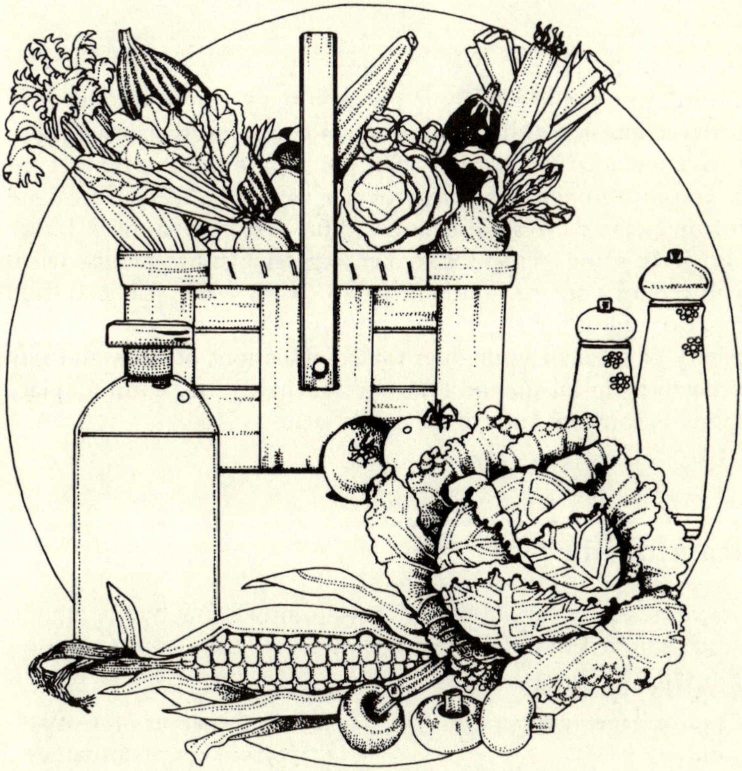

Many of the recipes in this chapter may be used as starters to a meal, just as some of those given in the previous chapter may be served as side dishes or light main courses in their own right. I have included this section because I believe salads, often served as accompaniments, are of particular value in a diet of this kind for they bring a fresh dimension to the texture of a meal. I have also given some recipes for cooked vegetable dishes because when you reduce your red-meat meals to two a week you may find that extra ideas for vegetables are useful. Of course, you will have plenty of ideas of your own for combinations of fresh and raw vegetables for salads, and I have not included such commonplace foods as coleslaw and mixed green salad.

Ratatouille

There are many variations of this well-known and, by my family, much enjoyed dish, but here is one.

500g/1lb courgettes
2 red or green peppers
1 onion
2ml/½ teaspoon salt
2ml/½ teaspoon rosemary
30ml/2 tablespoons SFS oil
1 aubergine
225g/8oz tomatoes or 1 small (225g/8oz) tin of tomatoes
2 cloves garlic
5ml/1 teaspoon basil
pepper

Heat the oil and add the diced onion and crushed garlic. Cut the courgettes and peppers in thin slices and cut the aubergine into small cubes. Add the vegetables to the onion and garlic. Stir well

to coat with the oil. Put the tomatoes through an electric blender and add these, with the herbs and seasoning, to the other vegetables, covering the pan. Simmer gently for about forty-five minutes. Ratatouille may be served as an accompaniment to a main-course dish or with low-fat cottage cheese as a light supper or lunch dish.
Fat: Nil
Oil: 40g/8 teaspoons

Fried Sprouting Beans

We produce our own sprouting beans in an American device in our sun lounge and find mung beans, aduki beans and soya beans all good for this dish. If you do not feel like producing your own beans they can be bought in tins.

2 onions
15ml/1 tablespoon SFS oil
pepper
100g/4oz sprouting beans
15ml/1 tablespoon soy sauce

Dice the onions finely and cook gently in the oil until transparent but not brown. Add the beans and stir constantly for about five minutes. Sprinkle with pepper and stir in the soy sauce before serving.
Fat: Nil
Oil: 20g/4 teaspoons

Mushroom and Cucumber Salad

Particularly delicious as a side salad served with pasta.

1 cucumber
15ml/1 tablespoon chopped fresh parsley
225g/8oz mushrooms

For the dressing

30ml/2 tablespoons SFS oil
2ml/½ teaspoon salt
30ml/2 tablespoons red wine vinegar

1 clove garlic
5ml/1 teaspoon French mustard
pepper

Without removing the skin of the cucumber, cut it into 6mm/¼in thick slices and each slice into four quarters. Cut the mushrooms into slices and mix with the cucumber and parsley. Put all the ingredients for the dressing into an electric blender and blend until smooth. Pour the dressing over the salad immediately before serving.
Fat: Nil
Oil: 40g/8 teaspoons

Orange and Green Pepper Salad

2 green peppers
2 oranges

For the dressing

1 clove garlic
30ml/2 tablespoons SFS oil
30ml/2 tablespoons orange juice
2ml/½ teaspoon salt

Remove the seeds from the peppers and cut into thin rounds. Peel the orange and cut it into thin slices at right angles to the lie of the segments. Arrange the pepper and orange rings in a serving dish. Put the ingredients for the dressing into an electric blender and blend until smooth. Pour over the salad immediately before serving.
Fat: Nil
Oil: 40g/8 teaspoons

White Cabbage Salad

Approx. 225g/8oz finely sliced white cabbage
25g/1oz chopped walnuts
French dressing (see p.22)
½ onion
2 cloves garlic
chopped fresh parsley to garnish

Crush the garlic with salt and mix it with the French dressing. Chop the onion finely. Mix the cabbage, onion and walnuts

together. Pour over the French dressing and toss well. Sprinkle the chopped parsley on to the salad before serving.
Fat: Nil
Oil: 60g/12 teaspoons

White Cabbage and Orange Salad

225g/8oz finely sliced white cabbage
25g/1oz raisins
2 oranges

For the dressing

15ml/1 tablespoon lemon juice
45ml/3 tablespoons SFS oil
2ml/½ teaspoon powdered cumin seed
salt and pepper

Make the dressing by shaking well together the lemon juice, oil and cumin powder. Season to taste.

Peel the oranges and cut the fruit in thin slices across the grain. Cut each slice into quarters. Mix the cabbage, orange and raisins and toss with the lemon dressing.
Fat: Nil
Oil: 60g/12 teaspoons

Spiced Red Cabbage

This dish is enjoyable hot or cold. It is very good served hot with jugged hare.

1 small red cabbage
30ml/2 tablespoons SFS oil
2 cooking apples
30–45ml/2–3 tablespoons red wine vinegar
100ml/4 fl oz water
2ml/½ teaspoon ground cloves
15ml/1 tablespoon brown sugar
salt and pepper

Quarter the cabbage and remove the central tough stalk. Slice the cabbage very finely. Peel, core and slice the apples finely. Put

all ingredients in a pan, bring to the boil and simmer very gently for about forty-five minutes.
Fat: Nil
Oil: 40g/8 teaspoons

Curried Cabbage

Another vegetable dish which is good hot or cold.

1 small cabbage (the firm white sort is best)
2 cloves garlic
15ml/1 tablespoon mango chutney
30ml/2 tablespoons water
1 onion
30ml/2 tablespoons SFS oil
10ml/2 teaspoons curry powder
salt

Chop the onion finely, crush the cloves of garlic and shred the cabbage very finely. Heat the oil in a large pan. Cook the onion and garlic gently in the oil until the onion is transparent but not brown. Add the curry powder and stir well. Add the rest of the ingredients and mix thoroughly. Cover with a tightly fitting lid and simmer gently for about seven minutes.
Fat: Nil
Oil: 40g/8 teaspoons

Chicory and Orange Salad

A delicious side salad with a meat or pasta dish.

2 heads chicory
French dressing made with 15ml/1 tablespoon SFS oil
2 oranges

Cut the chicory in thin slices. Peel the orange to remove all the pith. Cut the orange in slices across the grain of the segments and cut each slice into quarters. Mix the orange and chicory in individual dishes and pour over the dressing before serving.
Fat: Nil
Oil: 20g/4 teaspoons

Sweetcorn and Sweet Pepper Salad

1 green pepper
100g/4oz frozen sweetcorn
1 red pepper
French dressing made with 15ml/1 tablespoon SFS oil

Cook the corn until it is tender and allow it to cool. Slice the peppers finely and mix with the corn. Add the French dressing before serving.
Fat: Nil
Oil: 20g/4 teaspoons

Carrots in Orange Juice

This is most delicious made with new young carrots – we grow small round ones in a window box. It can also be prepared with sliced larger carrots or with frozen ones, but not with tinned carrots.

225g/8oz carrots
15ml/1 tablespoon soft light brown sugar
grated rind of ½ orange
60ml/4 tablespoons orange juice
25g/1oz PUF margarine
pinch ground mace
grated rind of ½ lemon
seasoning to taste

Mix all the ingredients together except the carrots and mix to a smooth syrup over a low heat. Add the carrots and simmer gently with the lid off the pan until the carrots are tender – this time will vary but with young ones will not be more than about ten minutes. Remove the carrots and put them in a serving bowl. Reduce the sauce until it is slightly caramelised and pour over the carrots. This dish can be served hot or cold.
Fat: 5g/1 teaspoon
Oil: Nil

Mushroom Salad

As with all the mushroom recipes given in this book, freshly picked and home-grown mushrooms give the best results.

225g/8oz mushrooms
30ml/2 tablespoons SFS oil
salt and pepper
2ml/½ teaspoon thyme
30ml/2 tablespoons lemon juice
5ml/1 teaspoon Dijon mustard
chopped fresh parsley to garnish

Slice the mushrooms. Mix together all the other ingredients except the chopped parsley. Put the mushrooms in a serving dish. Pour over the dressing. Garnish with the parsley before serving.
Fat: Nil
Oil: 40g/8 teaspoons

Green Pepper Medley

Finished in small ramekins, this is a good recipe for use as an accompaniment to a main course, but cooked in a larger casserole it is suitable for a lunch or supper dish.

1 onion
2 large green peppers
5ml/1 teaspoon basil
90ml/6 tablespoons dry white wine
100ml/4 fl oz skimmed milk
25g/1oz Parmesan cheese
15ml/1 tablespoon SFS oil
225g/8oz tomatoes or 1 small (225g/8oz) tin tomatoes
2 cloves garlic
30ml/2 tablespoons cornflour
salt and pepper

Heat the oil gently. Dice the onion, crush the garlic and cook both gently in the oil until the onion is transparent. Cut the peppers into small slices, add them to the pan and cook gently for about fifteen minutes or until they are tender. Add the cornflour and stir well. Remove the skins from the tomatoes and put the flesh in an electric blender. Add this or the tinned tomatoes to the pan with the wine and stir until the mixture boils. Add the milk, herbs and seasoning and simmer for a further five minutes. Put the mixture into one large serving dish or into ramekins, sprinkle with grated Parmesan cheese and brown under the grill.
Fat: 5g/1 teaspoon
Oil: 20g/4 teaspoons

Brown Rice Salad

Many variations can be made on this salad. I have given a fairly basic recipe and leave you to add the fish and meat which you fancy: this can include tuna, prawns, mussels, lean ham and chicken.

225g/8oz brown rice
½ green pepper
25g/1oz shredded white cabbage
salt
1 small onion
25g/1oz diced cucumber

For the dressing

30ml/2 tablespoons SFS oil
½ onion
2ml/½ teaspoon paprika
30ml/2 tablespoons cider vinegar
2 cloves garlic
5ml/1 teaspoon salt

Cook the brown rice for about thirty minutes in plenty of boiling salted water. Drain it and allow to cool. Chop the onion and green pepper finely and add them to the rice with the cabbage and diced cucumber. Put all the ingredients for the dressing through an electric blender until fairly smooth. Add the dressing to the rice and vegetables and stir well before serving.
Fat: Nil
Oil: 40g/8 teaspoons

Celery, Apple and Walnut Salad

Another crisp-textured side salad.

1 head celery
50g/2oz shelled walnuts (broken ones will do)
2 red-skinned eating apples
French dressing made with 15ml/1 tablespoon SFS oil

Wash the celery and cut into 6mm/¼in slices. Cut the apples into quarters, core them and cut into thin slices, leaving the skins on. Mix the celery, apple and walnuts and top with the dressing.
Fat: Nil
Oil: 20g/4 teaspoons

Fish

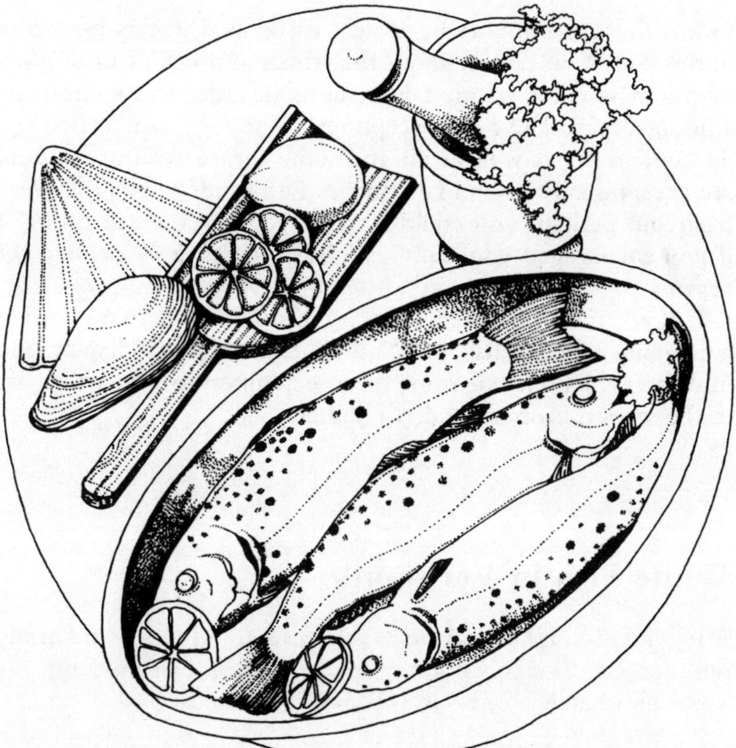

Fish is the most important protein to be used in this book and in this diet. You can eat about four times as much of most types of fish as you can of most lean meats in order to eat the same amount of fat. There are exceptions: some fish, such as herring, do contain fat as well as oil and some meats, such as venison, are exceptionally low in fat content. Fish needs to be eaten very fresh and perhaps you could increase your pleasure in eating it if you encouraged your family to learn to cast a fly or drag for prawns.

I have made a rather arbitrary distinction between dishes containing rice and fish, which are included in this chapter, and in dishes which include some meat in addition to fish, which are in the section on pasta and rice dishes.

White Fish in Vermouth

Any white fish fillets may be used for this dish. It is a wonderfully refreshing recipe for a hot day, or for somebody whose appetite is not good and who needs to be tempted to eat.

500g/1lb white fish fillets
60ml/4 tablespoons French vermouth
4 tablespoons water
peeled rind of 1 orange
chopped fresh parsley to garnish
salt and pepper

Season the fish. Put it in a fairly large shallow pan and cover with the vermouth, water and strips of orange peel. Allow to stand for an hour. Bring to the boil slowly and simmer very gently

for about ten minutes until the fish is well cooked. Remove the fish from the liquid and put it on a serving dish in a warm place. Remove the orange rind and boil the liquid fast and uncovered until it has halved its volume and become slightly thickened. Pour the juice over the fish and garnish with parsley before serving.
Fat: 10g/2 teaspoons
Oil: Nil

Telu's Fish Cutlets

A recipe given to me many years ago by a Pakistani who was a diplomat by profession and a cook by inclination.

500g/1lb or 12 cutlets of any white fish
15ml/1 tablespoon lemon juice
2ml/½ teaspoon ground ginger
2ml/½ teaspoon ground turmeric
125g/5oz home-made yoghurt
5ml/1 teaspoon salt
1 clove garlic
2ml/½ teaspoon chilli powder
2ml/½ teaspoon ground coriander seeds
15ml/1 tablespoon SFS oil

Mix the yoghurt with the lemon juice, spices and crushed clove of garlic. Add the fish cutlets and turn them several times. Leave them in the marinade for about six hours, turning once or twice. Remove them, paint lightly with SFS oil and cook under a hot grill until golden brown. This dish is excellent served with brown rice and a salad.
Fat: 10g/2 teaspoons
Oil: 20g/4 teaspoons

Kedgeree with Mushrooms and Peppers

500g/1lb smoked haddock fillets or a good-sized smoked haddock on the bone
30ml/2 tablespoons SFS oil
2 eggs
225g/8oz long-grain rice
salt and pepper
125g/5oz home-made yoghurt
1 green pepper
100g/4oz mushrooms
2 large onions
1 stick celery

Put the haddock in a covered pan with enough cold water to cover the fish. Bring to the boil and simmer until the fish is well cooked – about fifteen minutes. Remove the skin and bones (if any) and flake the remaining fish. Hard-boil the eggs. Allow them to cool and slice them. Chop the onions, pepper, celery and mushrooms finely. Heat the oil and add the onions, pepper and celery. Cook gently until the onion is transparent. Add the mushrooms and cook for another three or four minutes. Cook the rice for seventeen minutes in a large quantity of salted water. Strain and rinse well. Add the fish to the cooked vegetables and stir together. Then add the rice and the yoghurt and mix thoroughly over a low heat. Season to taste. Add the sliced hard-boiled eggs immediately before serving.
Fat: 20g/4 teaspoons
Oil: 40g/8 teaspoons

Island Turbot

1kg/2lb turbot off the bone
2 tomatoes
2 cloves garlic
2 bay leaves
30ml/2 tablespoons lemon juice
3 potatoes
1 onion
1 wine glass dry white wine
2ml/½ teaspoon thyme
salt and pepper

Wash and dry the fish and put it in an oven-to-table casserole. Slice the potatoes and onion very finely and arrange them round the fish. Cut the tomatoes in quarters, having removed the skins. Crush the cloves of garlic and mix together the tomatoes, garlic, seasoning, herbs, lemon juice and wine. Pour the mixture over the fish and bake in a moderate oven (180°C/350°F/gas mark 4) for about one and a quarter hours or until the vegetables are tender.
Fat: 40g/8 teaspoons
Oil: Nil

Trout Fried in Oatmeal

From the table where I am writing this I can see the burn, which is ours, and in which there are plenty of trout. It has been poached for so many years that nobody would now try to put an end to the practice; the result is there are no trout more than five inches long. One evening our son returned with eight trout of this size and I managed to get hold of them for long enough to try out this recipe before he ate five for his tea and the rest as a bed-time snack. It is a simple and excellent recipe done with reasonable-sized trout and preferably very fresh ones.

4 trout
45ml/3 tablespoons coarse oatmeal
60ml/4 tablespoons SFS oil
salt and pepper

Clean and fillet the trout. Mix the oatmeal with the salt and pepper. Heat the oil in a thick-bottomed pan. Dip each fillet in the oatmeal and fry in the oil, turning once, until each side is a golden brown. Serve with slices of lemon, new potatoes and a mixed green salad.
Fat: 20g/4 teaspoons
Oil: 80g/16 teaspoons

Psari Plaki

Oriental dishes – and this is one – are particularly useful in a low-fat diet as they provide many tasty ways of using fish, which in general is high in protein and low in fat; they are made traditionally using oil; and they can often be served with brown rice.

500g/1lb of any white fish cut into portions for serving
30ml/2 tablespoons SFS oil
350g/12oz of tomatoes or 1 500g/16oz can tomatoes without the juice
2 slices and the juice of 1 lemon
2 cloves garlic
1 large onion
125g/5oz dry white wine
salt and pepper
chopped fresh parsley to garnish

Chop the onion finely and crush the garlic. Heat the oil in a pan and brown the onion and garlic lightly. Skin and remove the pips from the tomatoes and add these to the pan together with the wine. Boil briskly without the lid on the pan until sufficiently reduced barely to cover the fish. Put the fish in the pan, put on the lid and simmer gently until the fish is tender. Add the seasoning and lemon juice. Serve garnished with a slice of lemon and chopped parsley. This dish is delicious served with boiled brown rice and a green salad tossed in French dressing.
Fat: 10g/2 teaspoons
Oil: 40g/8 teaspoons

Steamed Cod with Mustard Sauce

500g/1lb filleted white fish divided into four portions
salt and pepper
15ml/1 level tablespoon flour
chopped fresh parsley to garnish
skimmed milk to poach
15ml/1 tablespoon PUF margarine
5ml/1 teaspoon made mustard (English can be used but for a subtler flavour Dijon mustard is excellent)

Simmer the fish in enough milk to cover until cooked – this will take ten to fifteen minutes, depending on the thickness of the fillets. Lift the fish out of the pan, reserving the cooking liquid, and put in a serving dish in a warm place. Heat the margarine in another small pan and add the flour. Pour on the reserved cooking liquid and bring to the boil, stirring constantly. Add the mustard and blend in well. Adjust the seasoning. Pour the sauce over the fish and garnish with chopped fresh parsley.
Fat: 12·5g/2½ teaspoons
Oil: 30g/6 teaspoons

Prawn Curry

If you are able to obtain crayfish tails or other similar types of shellfish, they are excellent for this recipe. Made with fresh or frozen prawns, it is a delicious but expensive dish.

500g/1lb fresh or frozen prawns
2ml/½ teaspoon ground turmeric
5ml/1 teaspoon chilli powder
30ml/2 tablespoons SFS oil
1 onion
salt to taste
125g/5oz home-made yoghurt
2ml/½ teaspoon ground ginger
5ml/1 teaspoon ground cumin seeds
15ml/1 tablespoon lemon juice
4 cloves garlic

Chop the onion finely and crush the garlic and cook them in the oil until a medium brown. Add the spices and continue to cook for a further two minutes, stirring continuously. Add the yoghurt and cook very gently for ten minutes. Put in the prawns and the lemon juice and simmer very gently for another ten minutes. Serve with rice and any of the usual curry side dishes, such as sliced banana, sliced onion, grated apple and mango chutney.
Fat: 10g/2 teaspoons
Oil: 40g/8 teaspoons

Salmon Curry

Unfortunately salmon has a higher fat content than many other sorts of fish and a small helping is necessary to keep the fat intake down. I am including it because it is a particularly tasty and easily made dish. We fill up on lots of brown rice, a lentil puree and salad.

225g/8oz tin salmon
1 onion
10ml/2 teaspoons ground coriander seeds
5ml/1 teaspoon ground cumin seeds
salt to taste
4 cloves garlic
10ml/2 teaspoons ground turmeric
2ml/½ teaspoon ground ginger
2ml/½ teaspoon chilli powder
30ml/2 tablespoons SFS oil

Crush the garlic and dice the onion finely. Heat the oil and cook the onion and garlic in it until they are golden brown. Add the spices and continue to cook for a further five minutes, stirring continuously. Open the tin of salmon and gently put the contents in the pan. Break the fish into portions very carefully. Put a lid on the pan and simmer very gently for ten minutes. During this cooking time you must turn the pieces of salmon on several occasions without breaking them up.
Fat: 20g/4 teaspoons
Oil: 40g/8 teaspoons

Sole with Mushroom Sauce

Fillets of sole are delicious for this dish but it can be made with haddock or cod fillets. A wine glass of dry white wine may be added to the sauce and if this is done a little more cornflour should be used.

500g/1lb fillets of sole
100g/4oz mushrooms
salt and pepper
15ml/1 tablespoon cornflour
300ml/½ pint skimmed milk

Wash and dry the fish fillets and sprinkle them with salt and pepper. Reserving 30ml/2 tablespoons of milk, heat the rest in a large shallow pan to boiling point. Put in the fillets, lower the heat and poach them for five minutes. Take them out of the liquid and put them on a serving dish. Slice the mushrooms finely. Make a thin paste with the cornflour and 30ml/2 tablespoons of cold milk and pour on the milk in which the fish has cooked. Bring to the boil, stirring all the time. Add the finely sliced mushrooms and simmer for five minutes. Adjust the seasoning and pour the sauce over the fish before serving.
Fat: 10g/2 teaspoons
Oil: Nil

Grilled Salmon Steak with Hollandaise Sauce

As salmon is relatively high in fat, you will be having 5g/1 teaspoon of your day's fat allowance for every 50g/2oz of salmon that you eat. However, if you limit your steak to 100g/4oz you still have some margin.

4 × 100g/4oz salmon steaks
salt and pepper
15ml/1 tablespoon SFS oil

Brush the salmon steaks with oil on both sides and season lightly. Cook them under a heated grill for about six minutes on each side or until they are well done. Serve with Hollandaise sauce.

For the Hollandaise sauce

7ml/½ tablespoon SFS oil
15ml/1 tablespoon cornflour
100ml/4 fl oz water
1 egg yolk
¼ chicken stock cube
15ml/1 tablespoon lemon juice

Mix the oil and cornflour to a paste in a pan over a low heat. Add the water and the stock cube and bring to the boil, stirring constantly. Put the egg yolk and lemon juice in an electric blender and mix for a few seconds. Add the cornflour mixture and blend thoroughly.
Fat: 45g/9 teaspoons
Oil: 30g/6 teaspoons

Spanish Fish

Any white fish is good for this dish, including hake and cod.

4 white fish cutlets (about 500g/1lb)
50ml/2 fl oz skimmed milk
salt and pepper

For the sauce

4 large onions
30ml/2 tablespoons SFS oil
5ml/1 teaspoon mixed herbs
15ml/1 tablespoon tomato puree
6 cloves garlic
125ml/5 fl oz dry red wine
15ml/1 tablespoon lemon juice

Sprinkle the fish cutlets with salt and pepper on both sides and leave for twenty minutes. Simmer them gently in the skimmed milk in a covered pan for about fifteen minutes or until the fish is coming away from the bone. Put the cutlets in a serving dish and leave in a warm place.

To make the sauce: crush the cloves of garlic and dice the onions Heat the oil in a thick-bottomed pan and cook the onions and garlic very gently for twenty minutes with the lid on the pan. The onions should be well cooked but not browned. Put this mixture through an electric blender until it is quite smooth and then put it back in the pan. Add the wine, lemon juice, herbs and tomato puree. Simmer gently until the sauce thickens. Add salt and pepper if necessary. Pour the sauce over the fish and serve.

Fat: 10g/2 teaspoons
Oil: 40g/8 teaspoons

Fresh Haddock in White Wine and Curry

500g/1lb fillets cod or haddock
15ml/1 tablespoon curry powder
15ml/1 tablespoon SFS oil
2ml/½ teaspoon crushed fennel seeds
salt and pepper
125ml/5 fl oz dry white wine
1 large onion
15ml/1 tablespoon chopped fresh parsley
50g/2oz skimmed milk powder
30ml/2 tablespoons cold water

I use a flameproof casserole to make this dish because it saves washing up, though the first part of the cooking can, of course, be done in a pan and the rest in an oven-to-table casserole. Dice the onion and cook gently in the oil until it is transparent but not coloured. Cover with chopped parsley. Arrange the fish fillets on the parsley. Mix the wine, curry powder, crushed fennel seeds and seasoning together with a whisk and pour over the fish. Cook in a moderate oven, 180°C/350°F/gas mark 4, for thirty minutes. Mix the milk powder to a paste with the cold water and add to the fish and sauce before serving.

Fat: 10g/2 teaspoons
Oil: 20g/4 teaspoons

Trout Cooked in Paper

Trout is delicious cooked in this way but the recipe may be used for any small whole fish, such as haddock. I am estimating that each fish will be about 225g/8oz before preparation.

4 whole trout or other fish
30ml/2 tablespoons SFS oil
salt and pepper
4 large sheets greaseproof paper
4 sprigs parsley
4 wedges lemon

Gut and wash the fish, leaving the heads and tails on. Soak each piece of greaseproof paper in cold water. Paint each fish with SFS oil, season, add a sprig of parsley and wrap in a piece of paper, forming individual parcels. Twist the ends of the paper to make each parcel water-tight. Bring a large pan of water to the boil and put the four parcels into it. Boil gently for twelve minutes. Remove the parcels and serve the fish garnished with lemon wedges. This dish is delicious with new potatoes and fresh peas straight from the garden.
Fat: 15g/3 teaspoons (allowing for bones)
Oil: 40g/8 teaspoons

Mussel Salad

about 60 mussels
2 sticks celery
4 cloves garlic
1 potato
2ml/½ teaspoon fennel seeds
hearts of 2 lettuces
1 carrot
15ml/1 tablespoon tomato puree
100ml/4 fl oz dry white wine
15ml/1 tablespoon chopped fresh parsley
salt and pepper

Put the mussels to soak in a large bowl of cold water for several hours and change the water several times during this period: in this way the mussels will do a lot of the hard work by cleaning themselves. Discard any which are not tightly closed, take a small hard-bristled brush and brush off the 'beards'. Put the mussels into a large pan with the wine and cook them gently, shaking the pan frequently until all the shells open. This does not

take more than seven to ten minutes after the wine comes to the boil. Strain off the fish juice and wine and leave the mussels to cool. Put the liquid in another pan. Chop the carrot, celery and potato and crush the garlic and fennel seeds. Add these to the liquid and cook gently until tender – about twenty minutes. Add the tomato puree, and chopped parsley and season to taste. Put this mixture in an electric blender for a few seconds but do not let it get too smooth. Allow to cool. Arrange the broken hearts of the lettuce on a large serving dish. Spoon the vegetable mixture over and arrange the mussels on top. This makes an excellent light lunch or supper dish served with home-made brown bread.
Fat: 20g/4 teaspoons
Oil: Nil

Special Fish Pie

225g/8oz cod fillet
300ml/½ pint skimmed milk
225g/8oz smoked haddock fillet
1 bay leaf

For the sauce

15ml/1 tablespoon SFS oil
300ml/½ pint of the liquid from the cooked fish
1 egg
50g/2oz mushrooms
25g/1oz grated Parmesan cheese
15ml/1 tablespoon flour
15ml/1 tablespoon chopped parsley
500g/1lb smooth mashed potatoes

Simmer the fish in the milk with the bay leaf until it is tender – about twenty minutes. Strain off the liquid and keep 300ml/½ pint for the sauce. Remove the skin and bones from the fish and break it into small pieces. Warm the oil in a pan. Slice the mushrooms finely and cook gently in the oil for five minutes. Add the flour and stir well. Add the liquid and stir continuously until it comes to the boil. Boil gently for two minutes. Hard-boil the egg, slice it and add it with the parsley to the sauce. Mix the sauce and the fish and put them in an oven-to-table casserole.

Spread the mashed potatoes over the top, sprinkle with the Parmesan cheese and cook in a moderate oven 180°C/350°F/gas mark 4 for twenty-five minutes.
Fat: 20g/4 teaspoons
Oil: 20g/4 teaspoons

Coquilles St Jacques à la Provençale

This recipe has been given to me by the gourmet chef and owner of the Bridge Hotel at Bonar Bridge in Sutherland. He believes that it is impossible to run a hotel well unless the owner or manager has a profound knowledge of cooking, but he is becoming disillusioned because too many tourists are happiest with chips and beefburgers. If you happen to be passing on your way to John O' Groats, give him twenty-four hours' notice and he will produce a meal which you will remember with as much pleasure as my husband and I who have enjoyed many meals in this delightful hotel owned and run by Helen and Russell Taylor.

4 scallop shells
150g/6oz finely chopped onion
2 large cloves garlic (or to taste)
150ml/¼ pint liquor from scallops
salt and pepper
5ml/1 teaspoon mixed herbs
25g/1oz Parmesan cheese
10 scallops (frozen will do)
30ml/2 tablespoons SFS oil
150ml/¼ pint dry white wine
50g/2oz flour
1 bay leaf
225g/8oz smooth mashed potato

Put 15ml/1 tablespoonful of oil into a large frying pan and cook the onion, without colouring, with the pan covered. Add the garlic which has been crushed with salt, cook till transparent and then set aside. Slice the scallops 6mm/¼in thick. Dry the slices and dip in flour seasoned with salt and pepper. Put a tablespoonful of oil in the frying pan and fry the scallop slices until slightly coloured. Add the wine and liquor, bay leaf and mixed herbs and cook over a fast heat until the sauce thickens and reduces, stirring constantly to prevent sticking.

To prepare the shells, put the mashed potato into a forcing bag with a star tube and pipe around the edge of each shell. Pile

the cooked scallop mixture into the shells. Sprinkle with grated Parmesan cheese and grill until the cheese and potato are coloured.
Fat: 10g/2 teaspoons
Oil: 40g/8 teaspoons

Red Meat

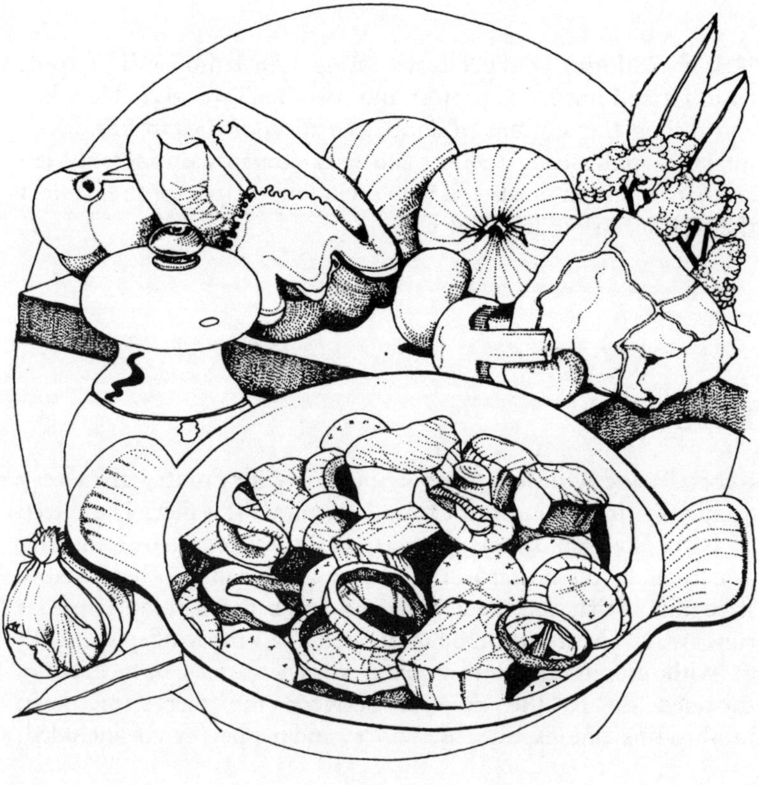

Half the calories you get from eating lean lamb or beef come from fat and not from protein and it is therefore advisable when controlling the amount of animal fat in your diet to limit your intake of red meat. Venison and hare contain considerably less fat than other red meats and I am including recipes for these under the section on poultry and game.

KEBABS

Kebabs made with lean lamb or beef or with poultry are a very good way of cooking meat for a low-animal-fat diet. They need to be cooked on kebab skewers about 25–30cm/10–12in long which can be placed across the base of a grill pan or other suitably sized tin so that the meat does not touch the base and any fat runs away. The meat can be marinated in a variety of spices, with or without yoghurt, and cooked with a variety of vegetables threaded on to the skewers between the pieces of meat: mushrooms, onions, tomatoes, celery and peppers can be included.

Spicy Lamb Kebabs

500g/1lb lean lamb from the leg
2 cloves garlic
5ml/1 teaspoon ground ginger
5ml/1 teaspoon ground cumin seeds
5ml/1 teaspoon salt
45ml/3 tablespoons home-made yoghurt
2 onions
10ml/2 teaspoons ground coriander seeds
5ml/1 teaspoon ground turmeric
1 large green pepper
50g/2oz button mushrooms
4 tomatoes

Cut the meat into 25mm/1in cubes. Crush the cloves of garlic and mix them with the yoghurt, spices and salt. Put the meat in this mixture and leave it, stirring occasionally, for at least four hours. Cut the onions into quarters, the tomatoes into quarters and the green pepper into 25mm/1in square pieces. Thread the kebab skewers with meat and pieces of vegetable to make an attractive display. Heat the grill and put the kebabs about 75mm/3in from the heat, cooking them for about eight minutes on each side. Serve with rice cooked with saffron and a mixed green salad.
Fat: 40g/8 teaspoons
Oil: Nil

Skewered Lamb with Mint Sauce

500g/1lb lean leg of lamb
10ml/2 teaspoons curry paste
5ml/1 teaspoon ground ginger
125g/5oz home-made yoghurt
15ml/1 tablespoon lemon juice

For the sauce

7ml/½ tablespoon chopped mint
5ml/1 teaspoon salt
2ml/½ teaspoon chilli powder
5ml/1 teaspoon sugar
1 small onion
30ml/2 tablespoons wine vinegar

Cut the lamb into 25mm/1in cubes. Mix together the yoghurt, curry paste, lemon juice and ground ginger and soak the meat in this mixture for at least twelve hours, stirring occasionally.

Remove the meat from the marinade and thread on to kebab skewers. Cook at a distance of about 75mm/3in from a very hot grill for about fifteen minutes, turning the skewers once. Put all the ingredients for the sauce into an electric blender until smooth. Serve the meat with brown rice, the prepared sauce and a mixed salad.
Fat: 40g/8 teaspoons
Oil: Nil

Lamb and Spring Vegetables

500g/1lb lean leg of lamb
500g/1lb new carrots
25g/1oz flour
a few sprigs fresh rosemary
2 sprigs fresh parsley
2 bay leaves
50g/2oz dried skimmed milk
1 onion
salt and pepper
500g/1lb fresh peas
300ml/½ pint skimmed milk
about 600ml/1 pint water
chopped fresh rosemary and parsley to garnish

Cut the lamb into 25mm/1in cubes. Slice the onion and put it with the meat and salt and pepper into a pan. Add the bay leaves, sprigs of rosemary and parsley and cover with water. Bring to the boil and simmer until tender which will be about an hour. Remove the sprigs of parsley and rosemary. Slice the carrots and add them to the lamb with the peas. Simmer for a further twenty minutes, checking that there is enough water. Mix the flour and dried skimmed milk with 45ml/3 tablespoons of the milk to a thin paste. Add the rest of the milk and stir into the meat and vegetable mixture. Bring back to the boil and cook for another five minutes before serving garnished with chopped parsley and rosemary.
Fat: 40g/8 teaspoons
Oil: Nil

Cassoulet

We find this dish so delicious in its original form with goose and belly of pork that we are prepared to enjoy it in this fat-reduced form. As there are many versions of this wonderful French dish I dare to produce one that is relatively low in animal fat.

500g/1lb white haricot beans
100g/4oz lean bacon in one piece
500g/1lb lean leg of lamb off the bone
15ml/1 tablespoon tomato puree
5ml/1 teaspoon thyme
15ml/1 tablespoon chopped fresh parsley
500g/1lb onions
30ml/2 tablespoons SFS oil
salt and pepper
6 cloves garlic
2 bay leaves

Soak the beans for at least twelve hours in cold water. Put them in a large pan with 2·4 litres/4 pints cold water and simmer covered for about two hours. Heat the oil in another large pan. Slice the onions. Brown the lamb, the piece of bacon and the sliced onions. Add the crushed cloves of garlic, tomato puree and herbs. Put 300ml/½ pint of the liquid in which the beans have cooked with the meat and herbs. Simmer for thirty minutes. Add the strained beans, keeping the rest of the liquid aside. Place the whole mixture in an oven-to-table casserole. Add enough of the bean liquid to cover all the ingredients. Cook in an oven at 180°C/350°F/gas mark 4 for about one and a half hours until the meat and beans are very tender. Adjust the seasoning and serve with boiled potatoes and a mixed green salad.
Fat: 50g/10 teaspoons
Oil: 40g/8 teaspoons

Beef and Lentil Curry

In this recipe the lentils increase the amount of protein in the dish without pushing up the amount of fat. There is ample for four helpings without resorting to the horror of a few bits of meat swimming in a large amount of curry sauce.

500g/1lb lean beef
2 onions
100g/4oz brown lentils
30ml/2 tablespoons SFS oil
5ml/1 teaspoon salt
2 cloves garlic
10ml/2 teaspoons curry powder
1ml/¼ teaspoon ground cloves
2ml/½ teaspoon ground cinnamon

Put the lentils in 1·2 litres/2 pints of cold water. Bring them to the boil and simmer until they are tender – about one and a half hours. Cut the beef into 25mm/1in cubes, crush the garlic and dice the onions. Heat the SFS oil in a pan and in it cook the onions and garlic until they are golden brown. Add the curry powder and spices and cook, stirring, for five minutes. Add the tomato puree and beef and continue cooking and stirring for a further five minutes. Strain 600ml/1 pint of the liquid in which the lentils have cooked on to the meat and simmer, covered, for about one hour until the meat is tender. Add the strained lentils and salt. Continue cooking without a cover on the pan until the lentils have disintegrated and the juice is thick. Serve with brown rice, grated raw vegetables and mango chutney.
Fat: 40g/8 teaspoons
Oil: 40g/8 teaspoons

Beef and Red Bean Casserole

The beans increase the amount of protein in this recipe and, if you want to make the dish more easily, may be bought tinned.

150g/6oz red kidney beans
500g/1lb lean beef
30ml/2 tablespoons SFS oil
600ml/1 pint water
2ml/½ teaspoon chopped thyme
2ml/½ teaspoon Tabasco sauce
1 green pepper
3 onions
30ml/2 tablespoons flour
½ beef stock cube
2ml/½ teaspoon oregano
5ml/1 teaspoon salt

Soak the beans overnight in cold water. Put them into fresh water, bring to the boil and simmer for one hour. Cut the meat into 25mm/1in cubes, slice the onions and deseed and slice the pepper finely. Heat the SFS oil in a heavy pan and fry the onions and pepper gently until the onions are golden. Turn up the heat and brown the meat, stirring constantly. Add the flour and cook for a further two minutes while stirring. Add the water and stock cube and stir until the mixture boils. Add the drained beans, herbs, Tabasco sauce and salt. Cover the pan and simmer gently for about one and a half to two hours until the meat is tender.

Fat: 40g/8 teaspoons
Oil: 40g/8 teaspoons

Leg of Lamb with Wine Sauce

The total amount of fat in this recipe will look a great deal but the dish should be regarded either as a party dish or one that will last for several days; this can be especially useful in school holidays or when there are guests around.

2kg/4lb leg of lamb
3 cloves garlic
1 carrot
15ml/1 tablespoon SFS oil
15ml/1 tablespoon flour
½ bottle red wine
2 onions
10ml/2 teaspoons mixed herbs
1 bay leaf
salt and pepper

Mix the wine, herbs, bay leaf, crushed garlic, sliced onions and carrot and salt and pepper. Put the leg of lamb in a tin or dish just large enough to hold it and pour the wine mixture over it. Put in a cool place and leave to marinate for twenty-four hours, or longer if possible, turning the joint several times during this period. Remove the meat from the marinade, put it in a roasting tin and cook in the oven for one hour at 200°C/400°F/ gas mark 6. Bring the wine and vegetables to the boil and simmer for twenty minutes or until the vegetables are tender. Put the mixture through an electric blender until it is quite smooth. Heat the SFS oil in a clean pan, add the flour and mix well. Add the blended wine mixture, bring to the boil and simmer for two minutes. Serve the sauce with the meat. Both the meat and the sauce can be eaten hot or cold.

Fat: 120g/24 teaspoons
Oil: 20g/4 teaspoons

Lamb Stewed with Red Wine

500g/1lb lean lamb cut from the leg or flank
225g/8oz mushrooms
50g/2oz lean bacon
30ml/2 tablespoons SFS oil
15ml/1 tablespoon chopped fresh parsley
2ml/½ teaspoon thyme
salt and pepper
300ml/½ pint red wine
225g/8oz small onions
30ml/2 tablespoons flour
5ml/1 teaspoon rosemary
1 bay leaf
300ml/½ pint water

Cut the lamb into 40mm/1½in cubes and dice the bacon. Peel the onions. Heat the oil in a heavy pan and add the lamb, bacon and onions and fry them until golden brown on all sides. Add the flour and stir in well. Add the wine and water and continue stirring until it comes to the boil. Add the herbs and seasoning. Cover and simmer for about one hour. Add the mushrooms and simmer for a further fifteen minutes.
Fat: 40g/8 teaspoons
Oil: 20g/4 teaspoons

Calf's Liver in Wine

500g/1lb calf's liver
1 wine glass red wine
7ml/½ tablespoon chopped fresh parsley
5ml/1 teaspoon tarragon
15ml/1 tablespoon flour
30ml/2 tablespoons SFS oil
15ml/1 tablespoon brandy
5ml/1 teaspoon chopped chives
salt and pepper

Cut the liver into eight pieces of even size. Heat the SFS oil in a pan and fry the liver on each side until lightly cooked. Remove the liver and put it in a serving dish. Sprinkle the flour into the pan and stir well for one minute. Add the brandy, red wine, herbs and seasoning, bring back to the boil, stirring continuously, and simmer for two minutes. Pour the sauce over the liver. This dish is good served with brown rice and a mixed or tomato salad.
Fat: 15g/3 teaspoons
Oil: 40g/8 teaspoons

Lamb Curry

500g/1lb lean lamb, preferably from the leg
4 onions
30ml/2 tablespoons SFS oil
2ml/½ teaspoon ground coriander seeds
2ml/½ teaspoon ground cumin seeds
5ml/1 teaspoon salt
4 cloves garlic
5ml/1 teaspoon ground turmeric
2ml/½ teaspoon ground ginger
2ml/½ teaspoon chilli powder
450ml/¾ pint water

Cut the lamb into 25mm/1in cubes. Slice the onions finely and crush the garlic. Heat the oil in a pan and cook the onions and garlic until they are brown. Add all the spices and cook, stirring continuously, for four minutes. Add the cubes of meat and continue to cook, turning the meat from time to time, for another six minutes. Add the water and salt, bring back to the boil, cover and simmer for one hour. This curry should have very little juice and it may be necessary to finish the cooking without the cover on the pan. Serve with boiled rice and the usual accompaniments.
Fat: 40g/8 teaspoons
Oil: 40g/8 teaspoons

Kidneys with Apple

500g/1lb lamb's or calf's kidneys without the fat
15ml/1 tablespoon flour
30ml/2 tablespoons SFS oil
30ml/2 tablespoons cider
225g/8oz brown rice
2 large cooking apples
salt and pepper
30ml/2 tablespoons lemon juice

Peel, core and thinly slice the apples. Heat the oil in a pan until fairly hot and fry the apples until they are brown on both sides, turning them once but not allowing them to lose their shape. Drain the apple slices on greaseproof paper. Mix the flour with the salt and pepper. Core the kidneys, cut into thin slices and mix well with the seasoned flour. Put the meat in the oil and cook for about twelve minutes, turning the pieces at frequent intervals. Add the cider and lemon juice, stirring continuously until the sauce thickens. Meanwhile cook the brown rice in salted water for twenty-five to thirty minutes, then drain. Arrange the apple rings at an angle around the edge of a round or oval bowl. Put the cooked rice in the bottom of the bowl and pour the kidneys and sauce over the rice but not over the apple. Serve with a green salad.

Fat: 15g/3 teaspoons
Oil: 40g/8 teaspoons

Barbecued Lamb with Mint and Honey

This recipe produces an alarming figure for the total quantity of fat but, as with lamb and wine sauce, it will do for a party or last a family for a number of meals. You will need a method of rotisserie cooking for this dish.

2kg/4lb leg of lamb
salt and pepper
2 cloves garlic

For the glaze

30ml/2 tablespoons SFS oil
30ml/2 tablespoons prepared mint jelly
30ml/2 tablespoons honey

Dry the leg of lamb. Cut the cloves of garlic into slivers and insert them with the point of a sharp knife at different places in the lamb. Season the joint with salt and pepper. Insert the spit and holding prongs according to the instructions given. Heat the oven to 160°C/325°F/gas mark 3, put in the meat and cook it for one and a half hours. Mix together all the ingredients for the glaze. Baste the lamb with the glaze after it has cooked for one hour.

Fat: 120g/24 teaspoons
Oil: 40g/8 teaspoons

Poultry and Game

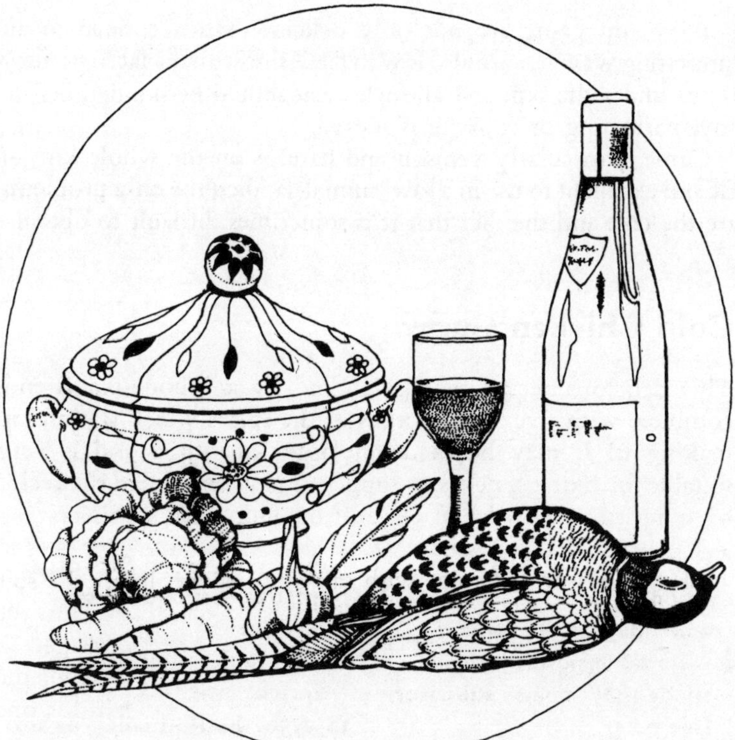

Poultry and game are not only delicious when cooked in an interesting way, but are also low in fat. Almost all the fat in poultry is just under the skin and all such meat should be skinned before any marinating or cooking is started.

Game, particularly venison and hare, is on the whole low in fat and excellent to use in a low-animal-fat diet; the only problems are the cost and the fact that it is sometimes difficult to obtain.

Cold Chicken Curry

This delicious recipe was given me by a Rhodesian friend, complete with five small bottles of the spices which she uses in making it. It may be made in larger quantities and is very suitable for buffet lunches or suppers. I have simplified the recipe by using curry powder in place of the individual spices.

1 cold boiled chicken
1 onion
1 wine glass white wine
90ml/6 tablespoons home-made mayonnaise substitute (see p.24)
salt and pepper
15ml/1 tablespoon SFS oil
15ml/1 tablespoon curry powder
15ml/1 tablespoon smooth apricot jam
125g/5oz home-made yoghurt

Remove the skin from the chicken and break the flesh into bite-sized portions. Mix all the other ingredients together. Add the chicken. Leave in a cool place overnight if possible as the flavour improves with standing.

Fat: 40g/8 teaspoons
Oil: 20g/4 teaspoons

Tandoori Chicken

4 chicken joints, skinned
30ml/2 tablespoons lemon juice
15ml/1 tablespoon SFS oil
5ml/1 teaspoon chilli powder
2 cloves garlic
125g/5oz home-made yoghurt
5ml/1 teaspoon salt
2ml/½ teaspoon ground ginger
5ml/1 teaspoon ground coriander seeds

Mix the yoghurt, lemon juice, spices, salt and crushed cloves of garlic. Put the chicken in this marinade and leave for at least twelve hours, turning the joints from time to time. Heat the grill. Drain the chicken joints and paint them with SFS oil. Cook them under a hot grill until very well cooked. Serve with saffron rice and a tomato salad garnished with onion rings.

Fat: 20g/4 teaspoons
Oil: 20g/4 teaspoons

Chicken Provençal

If you use a whole chicken this dish will be sufficient for six people, but use four chicken joints if you need only enough for the family. A delicious dish for a Sunday lunch or a buffet supper.

4 chicken joints, skinned
1 onion
1 small green pepper
2 cloves garlic
15ml/1 tablespoon concentrated tomato puree
450ml/¾ pint liquid made from a mixture of dry white wine and water (the proportion can be varied to suit your taste)
5ml/1 teaspoon rosemary
15ml/1 tablespoon chopped fresh parsley
salt and pepper
30ml/2 tablespoons SFS oil
225g/8oz tomatoes or 1 small (225g/8oz) tin tomatoes
150g/6oz mushrooms
5ml/1 teaspoon basil
1ml/¼ teaspoon thyme

Brown the chicken joints in the heated oil and then remove them from the pan. Chop the onion finely and brown in the hot oil. Chop the green pepper after removing the seeds and remove the tomato skins if using fresh tomatoes. Put the chicken back into the pan, add the vegetables, liquid, tomato puree, herbs and

seasoning. Cover the pan and simmer for one and a half hours, adding the mushrooms for the last half-hour. Remove the chicken joints and vegetables. Reduce the liquid until of the required consistency. Pour over the chicken joints and serve. This is delicious served with brown rice and a green salad with French dressing.
Fat: 40g/8 teaspoons
Oil: 40g/8 teaspoons

Pastel del Choclo

A delicious Chilean chicken dish for which my husband acquired a liking while he was working in Chile. The recipe was given me by a friend who is a native of that country. It is often served as a party dish and I have reduced the amount of ingredients so that the quantity is suitable for a family.

100g/4oz minced lean beef
1 large onion
10ml/2 teaspoons basil
30ml/2 tablespoons SFS oil
350g/12oz frozen sweetcorn kernels
15ml/1 tablespoon icing sugar
salt and pepper
4 small chicken joints, skinned
2ml/½ teaspoon thyme
1ml/¼ teaspoon mixed spice
1 hard-boiled egg
90ml/6 tablespoons prepared skimmed dried milk
25g/1oz raisins

Chop the onion finely and fry until golden brown in 1 tablespoon SFS oil. Add the minced beef, herbs, mixed spice and salt and pepper. Line the base of an oven-to-table pie dish with this mixture. Slice the hard-boiled egg and put the slices over the meat mixture. Sprinkle with raisins and arrange the chicken joints as the next layer. Thaw the frozen corn and simmer gently with the milk, basil, 1 tablespoon SFS oil and some salt until tender. Put through a blender until creamy. Pour the corn over the top of the pie, sprinkle with icing sugar and bake in an oven at 180°C/350°F/gas mark 4 for forty minutes or until the corn is golden brown.
Fat: 35g/7 teaspoons
Oil: 40g/8 teaspoons

Chicken with Turmeric and Rice

1 chicken
1 small (225g/8oz) tin tomatoes
2 cloves garlic
225g/8oz long-grain rice
salt and pepper
2 onions
30ml/2 tablespoons SFS oil
600ml/1 pint water
15ml/3 teaspoons turmeric
5ml/1 teaspoon basil

Remove the skin from the chicken. Chop the onions finely. Heat 1 tablespoon SFS oil in a large pan and cook half the chopped onion in it until transparent but not coloured. Turn up the heat, put in the chicken and turn it so that it browns on all sides. Turn down the heat and add the seasoning, tomatoes, basil, 7·5ml/1½ teaspoons of the turmeric and the crushed cloves of garlic. Simmer very gently for about one hour until the chicken is tender. Soften the other half of the chopped onion in the other tablespoon of SFS oil. Stir in the rice and the remaining 7·5ml/1½ teaspoons of turmeric and continue to stir until all the oil is absorbed and the turmeric is evenly distributed. Add the water and simmer for about twenty minutes until all the liquid is absorbed. Put the cooked chicken in a serving dish, pour the liquid over it and serve the rice separately.
Fat: 40g/8 teaspoons
Oil: 40g/8 teaspoons

Chicken Curry

Using individual spices it is possible to adapt the flavour of this and other curries to suit the palate of your family. How hot the curry is depends on the amount of ground chilli that you put in. As I do for my family, you may need to make two batches of this curry – one hot and the other not so hot.

4 chicken joints, skinned
2 onions chopped finely
1ml/¼ teaspoon ground cloves
3 cloves garlic, crushed with salt
30ml/2 tablespoons SFS oil
1ml/¼ teaspoon ground cardamom
2ml/½ teaspoon ground cumin seeds

2ml/½ teaspoon turmeric
2ml/½ teaspoon ground ginger
1–2ml/¼–½ teaspoon ground chilli, according to taste
½ stick cinnamon
10ml/2 teaspoons ground coriander seeds
300ml/½ pint water

Put the SFS oil in a thick-bottomed pan with a lid. Fry the onions, garlic and spices until the onions are a golden brown. Add the chicken joints and continue to fry for at least ten minutes, stirring frequently. Add the water, put the lid on the pan and cook slowly until the chicken is tender and there is a concentrated sauce. Serve the chicken with brown rice and a green salad as well as some of the usual accompaniments, such as sliced banana and mango chutney.
Fat: 40g/8 teaspoons
Oil: 40g/8 teaspoons

Chicken in Yoghurt and Wine Sauce

4 small chicken joints, skinned
1 onion
15ml/1 tablespoon flour
½ chicken stock cube
100g/4oz mushrooms
salt and pepper
30ml/2 tablespoons SFS oil
300ml/½ pint water
100g/4oz home-made yoghurt
grated rind of 1 lemon
½ wine glass dry white wine

Slice the onion finely and skin the chicken joints. Heat the oil in a pan and cook the onion until soft. Remove from the pan, then cook the chicken until it is golden brown. Return the onion to the pan, add the flour and stir until the flour and oil are a light brown. Add the water, chicken stock cube and seasoning, cover the pan and simmer gently for thirty minutes. Add the sliced mushrooms and simmer for a further ten minutes. Remove the chicken joints. Add the yoghurt, white wine and lemon rind. Bring back to the boil and simmer uncovered until of a creamy consistency. Adjust the seasoning and pour the sauce over the chicken joints.
Fat: 20g/4 teaspoons
Oil: 40g/8 teaspoons

Chicken Maryland

4 chicken breasts, skinned
15ml/1 tablespoon flour
salt and pepper
2 bananas
30ml/2 tablespoons SFS oil
breadcrumbs and skimmed milk for frying

Mix the flour with the salt and pepper. Dip the chicken breasts in the flour and then into the skimmed milk and breadcrumbs. Using a fairly small frying pan, heat the oil and fry the chicken pieces until brown on both sides. Cover the pan and cook gently for another twenty minutes or until the chicken is well cooked. Remove the chicken pieces and drain them on greaseproof paper.

Split the bananas lengthwise and cut each slice across the middle. Heat the oil again and fry the bananas until brown on both sides.

For the sweetcorn fritters

50g/2oz cooked sweetcorn
salt and pepper
15ml/1 tablespoon flour
15ml/1 tablespoon skimmed milk
watercress to garnish

Mix together the cooked corn, milk, flour and seasoning. Form into four flat rounds, dip into skimmed milk and breadcrumbs and fry in the same fat as the bananas until brown on both sides. Arrange the chicken joints, bananas and sweetcorn fritters on a serving dish and garnish with watercress before serving.
Fat: 20g/4 teaspoons
Oil: 40g/8 teaspoons

Chicken with Tomatoes and Peppers

500g/1lb chicken meat from the breast and the leg
30ml/2 tablespoons cornflour
30ml/2 tablespoons SFS oil
1 large (500g/16oz) tin tomatoes
2 green peppers
2 cloves garlic
5ml/1 teaspoon ground ginger
salt and pepper
15ml/1 tablespoon soy sauce
4 onions
30ml/2 tablespoons sherry
300ml/½ pint water
½ chicken stock cube

Skin the chicken and cut the flesh into 50mm/2in portions. Dice the onions, slice the peppers and crush the garlic. Mix together the sherry and soy sauce and dip the chicken portions in this mixture and then in the seasoned cornflour. Fry for about six minutes in the heated oil, turning once, until the pieces are brown on both sides. Remove them from the oil and drain. Add the onions, peppers and garlic and cook gently until the onions are transparent but not coloured. Add the tomatoes, ginger, water and stock cube, bring to the boil and simmer for ten minutes in an uncovered pan. Reduce the sauce if necessary by turning up the heat for a few minutes. Pour over the chicken slices.
Fat: 20g/4 teaspoons
Oil: 40g/8 teaspoons

Chicken Paprika

4 small chicken joints, skinned
60ml/4 tablespoons water
salt and pepper
5ml/1 teaspoon paprika
450ml/¾ pint chicken stock
50g/2oz dried skimmed milk
15ml/1 tablespoon lemon juice
15ml/1 tablespoon SFS oil
1 onion
15ml/1 tablespoon tomato puree
15ml/1 tablespoon flour

Dice the onion and cook gently in the heated oil until transparent but not brown. Add the paprika and stir well for one minute. Add 100ml/4 fl oz of the chicken stock and the chicken joints to the pan. Cover and simmer for about forty minutes until the chicken is tender. Remove the chicken joints from the liquid. Add the tomato puree and the rest of the chicken stock to the pan and bring back to the boil. Put the skimmed-milk powder and the flour together in a bowl and mix to a paste with the 4 tablespoons of water. Pour part of the boiling liquid on to the mixture, stir well and then return to the pan. Stir the liquid until it has come to the boil, adjust the seasoning and simmer for five minutes. Pour this sauce over the chicken pieces and serve.
Fat: 20g/4 teaspoons
Oil: 20g/4 teaspoons

Mediterranean Chicken

4 chicken joints
1 small (225g/8oz) tin tomatoes
30ml/2 tablespoons flour
300ml/½ pint chicken stock
15ml/1 tablespoon tomato puree
1 onion
2 stalks celery
30ml/2 tablespoons SFS oil
2 cloves garlic
1 small carrot
1 wine glass white wine
salt and pepper
100g/4oz button mushrooms
chopped fresh parsley to garnish

Heat the oil, remove the skin from the chicken joints and cook them slowly on both sides until golden brown. Remove them from the fat and put them in a serving dish. Dice the onion, crush the garlic, chop the carrot and celery and add these to the fat and fry until the vegetables begin to change colour. Sprinkle the flour over and cook, stirring, for three minutes. Add the tomato puree, tomatoes, wine, chicken stock and seasoning. Bring to the boil and simmer for twenty minutes. Put this mixture through an electric blender until it is smooth. Return it to the pan and add the mushrooms. Simmer for ten minutes with the pan uncovered and then pour the sauce and mushrooms over the chicken joints. Garnish with the chopped parsley before serving.
Fat: 20g/4 teaspoons
Oil: 40g/8 teaspoons

GAME

We are fortunate enough to rent some shooting and have a son who is a good shot. At times I am amply supplied with hares, grouse, partridge and duck but at others such hazards as bad weather, too many examinations or the partridge left to hang over the plastic container full of engine oil from a motor bike and snapping its moorings can make the supply erratic. If you can get hare, rabbit and venison they are all valuable meats because they are low in fat.

Venison Casserole

1kg/2lb shoulder of venison
30ml/2 tablespoons SFS oil
2 onions
1 bay leaf
15ml/1 tablespoon redcurrant jelly
2 cloves garlic
450ml/$\frac{3}{4}$ pint red wine
30ml/2 tablespoons flour
2 carrots
5ml/1 teaspoon mixed herbs
salt and pepper

Slice the onions and the carrots and crush the cloves of garlic and put these into a dish with the red wine. Cut the venison into 40mm/1$\frac{1}{2}$in cubes and put the meat into the marinade and leave for twenty-four to thirty-six hours. Remove the pieces of meat, dry them and cook in the heated oil, turning them until they are sealed on all sides. Sprinkle the flour over the meat and stir until it is browned and well mixed in. Add the marinade and seasoning, herbs and bay leaf. Bring to the boil, cover the pan and simmer for at least two hours or until the meat is tender. Put the meat in a serving dish; reduce the sauce if necessary, remove the bay leaf, stir in the redcurrant jelly and pour over the meat.
Fat: 20g/4 teaspoons
Oil: 40g/8 teaspoons

Braised Venison

1kg/2lb haunch of venison
15ml/1 tablespoon SFS oil
6 juniper berries
2 carrots
15ml/1 tablespoon redcurrant jelly
30ml/2 tablespoons flour
1 bay leaf
300ml/$\frac{1}{2}$ pint red wine
a few sprigs parsley and marjoram
3 onions
2 stalks celery
salt and pepper
300ml/$\frac{1}{2}$ pint water

Slice one onion and put it with the bay leaf, crushed juniper berries and herb sprigs in the red wine. Put the joint of venison in this marinade and leave for at least twelve hours, turning it over from time to time. Put the oil to heat in a flame-proof ovenware dish. Dice the other two onions, slice the carrots and celery. Put the joint of venison in the pan and brown quickly on both sides.

Remove it and put in the vegetables, stir them for about two minutes, pour off the excess oil and replace the joint of venison on top of the vegetables. Strain the wine from the marinade over the meat and add the water and seasoning. Cover the casserole and put it in a slow oven at 150°C/300°F/gas mark 2 for two hours. Remove the meat, carve it, put it on a serving dish and keep warm. Put the flour, the juice and vegetables from the braising pan and the redcurrant jelly into an electric blender and blend until smooth. Return to the pan, bring to the boil and simmer for two minutes. Pour over the venison before serving.
Fat: 20g/4 teaspoons
Oil: 20g/4 teaspoons

Country Pigeons

Pigeons are not exactly game and they are a nuisance to prepare but if you can get them, preferably ready prepared, this is an excellent dish.

4 pigeons
225g/8oz pickling onions
150g/6oz button mushrooms
1 wine glass white wine
5ml/1 teaspoon sugar
100g/4oz lean bacon in one piece
15ml/1 tablespoon SFS oil
15ml/1 tablespoon flour
600ml/1 pint chicken stock

Heat the oil in a large pan. Cut the bacon into small cubes and cook until it is a golden brown on all sides. Remove it and put it in an ovenware casserole. Skin the onions and brown them in the fat, sprinkling them with the teaspoon of sugar. Remove and put them with the bacon. Brown the pigeons on all sides and put them also in the casserole. Add the flour to the oil and cook, stirring, for one minute. Add the wine and stock slowly, stirring all the time, bring back to the boil and simmer for two minutes. Strain the sauce over the pigeons, cover the casserole and cook it in a very moderate oven 160°C/325°F/gas mark 3 for one and a half hours or until the pigeon meat is beginning to come away from the bone. Add the mushrooms half an hour before the cooking is finished.
Fat: 20g/4 teaspoons
Oil: 20g/4 teaspoons

Rabbit in Red Wine

1 large rabbit
225g/8oz button mushrooms
30ml/2 tablespoons SFS oil
300ml/½ pint chicken stock
5ml/1 teaspoon salt
pepper
100g/4oz whole small onions
15ml/1 tablespoon flour

For the marinade

300ml/½ pint red wine
1 medium onion
1 bay leaf
2ml/½ teaspoon allspice
5ml/1 teaspoon thyme

Slice the medium onion and add with the bay leaf, thyme and allspice to the red wine. Joint the rabbit and put the pieces in the wine marinade. Leave them for at least twelve hours, turning them from time to time. Heat the oil in a large pan. Remove the rabbit joints from the marinade and brown them in the oil. Take the joints out of the oil and put them in an ovenware casserole. Skin the 100g/4oz onions, add them whole to the pan and cook until they are golden brown. Remove them and put them with the rabbit. Sprinkle the flour into the pan and cook, stirring, for two minutes. Add the strained marinade, the chicken stock and the seasoning. Bring to the boil, stirring all the time, and simmer for two minutes. Pour over the rabbit. Put a lid on the casserole and cook it in a moderate oven (180°C/350°F/gas mark 4) for one hour. Add the mushrooms after half an hour. Adjust the seasoning before serving.
Fat: 20g/4 teaspoons
Oil: 40g/8 teaspoons

Partridge Casserole

2 partridges
3 onions
5ml/1 teaspoon mixed herbs
15ml/1 tablespoon flour
600ml/1 pint water
50g/2oz lean bacon in one piece
150g/6oz button mushrooms
1 wine glass red wine
30ml/2 tablespoons SFS oil
salt and pepper
chopped fresh parsley to garnish

Heat the oil in a large pan and brown the prepared partridges in the hot oil. Remove the partridges and keep them warm. Dice the onions and the bacon and put them in the fat. When they are golden brown, sprinkle the flour over them and stir for two minutes. Add the wine, water, seasoning and mixed herbs. Bring back to the boil and turn down to simmering point. Replace the partridges and cook over a low heat for about two hours or until the flesh of the partridges is very tender. Add the mushrooms after about one and a half hours. Take the partridges out of the sauce and cut each bird in half. Put the halves in a serving dish. Remove the mushrooms from the pan and reduce the sauce to the desired consistency before replacing the mushrooms in it, pouring it over the partridges and garnishing with the chopped parsley.

Fat: 15g/3 teaspoons
Oil: 40g/8 teaspoons

Jugged Hare

If you are able to be fussy about your hare, choose a hill or blue hare rather than the larger brown variety. It will need hanging and cooking a little longer but the flavour is better.

1 hare, prepared and cut into pieces
2 large onions
30ml/2 tablespoons SFS oil
5ml/1 teaspoon allspice
1 stalk celery
15ml/1 tablespoon lemon juice
15ml/1 tablespoon redcurrant jelly
15ml/1 tablespoon flour
2 whole cloves
5ml/1 teaspoon mixed herbs
1 carrot
salt and pepper
900ml/1½ pints water
the blood from the hare

For the marinade

150ml/¼ pint red wine
2 bay leaves
1 onion
4 juniper berries
15ml/1 tablespoon SFS oil
salt and pepper

Slice the onion and boil all the ingredients for the marinade together for about one minute. Cool and pour over the pieces of hare. Leave for twenty-four hours, turning the hare at intervals.

Heat the oil and brown the pieces of hare in it. Stick one clove into each of the onions and slice the carrot and celery. Put the pieces of hare and vegetables into a casserole. Sprinkle the flour over the fat and stir until it is brown. Add the water, herbs, spice and seasoning and bring the mixture to the boil. Simmer for two minutes and pour over the hare and vegetables in the casserole. Cover the casserole and cook for three hours in an oven at 150°C/300°F/gas mark 2. Add the lemon juice and redcurrant jelly about half an hour before the end of the cooking time. Remove the hare and the vegetables and place in a serving dish. Put the remainder of the juice with the strained marinade and blood from the hare in a pan on the top of the stove and simmer uncovered until it is the consistency of thin cream. Strain it over the joints of hare and serve with boiled potatoes and freshly cooked brussel sprouts or a red cabbage salad.

Fat: 30g/6 teaspoons
Oil: 40g/8 teaspoons

Pheasant with Red Wine

2 young pheasants
150ml/¼ pint red wine
50g/2oz thinly sliced lean bacon
salt and pepper

Put the pheasants in a casserole just large enough to hold them. Arrange the slices of bacon over the pheasants. Season the birds, pour the wine over them and cover the dish. Cook for one and a quarter hours in an oven at 180°C/350°F/gas mark 4. This is good served with boiled brown rice, braised celery and a side salad.

Fat: 20g/4 teaspoons
Oil: Nil

Pasta and Rice Dishes

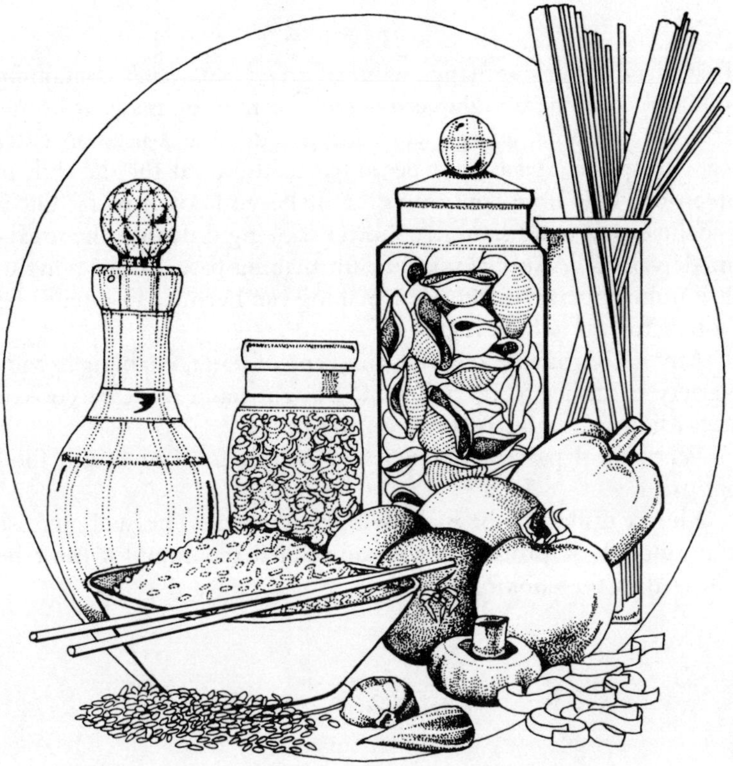

Pasta in all its various shapes, white or green (*pasta verdi*, containing spinach), may be bought ready-made or may be made at home. If made at home, an egg yolk can be added and if so an extra 5g/1 teaspoon of fat must be added to the total for the dish in question. It is time-consuming to make your own pasta, but it is delicious; it will also need a shorter cooking time than the ready-made variety. A special machine for making pasta can be bought. It is quite expensive, but pasta-making can become an interesting hobby for the whole family.

Any sauce may be used for any type of pasta, enabling a wide variety of dishes to be prepared. Bought pasta must be cooked according to the instructions on the packet.

Wholemeal pasta is obtainable at whole food or health food shops.

All rice dishes can be made with brown rice. This will increase the amount of protein but an additional ten minutes must be allowed in the cooking time.

Paella

This dish is more than enough for a family of four but can be useful for a buffet supper or lunch.

4 small chicken joints, skinned
2 onions
3 cloves garlic
1 small (225g/8oz) tin tomatoes
900ml/1½ pints chicken stock
45ml/3 tablespoons SFS oil
225g/8oz prawns
2 green peppers
350g/12oz long-grain rice
salt and pepper
50g/2oz cooked peas

Heat the oil in a large heavy-bottomed pan or in a special paella pan if you have one. Dice the onions and crush the garlic, and cook them in the oil until the onions are soft but not coloured. Cut each chicken joint into two or three pieces and put them into the pan. Cook them until they have coloured on both sides. Deseed and finely slice the green peppers, add to the pan and cook, stirring the contents, for a further five minutes. Add the rice and continue stirring for another five minutes. Add the tin of tomatoes, the chicken stock and seasoning, bring back to the boil and simmer with the pan uncovered for about twenty minutes until the rice is tender and all the fluid is absorbed. Stir from time to time. Add the cooked prawns and peas and stir, allowing them to heat through. Turn the heat to very low until you are ready to serve the dish.
Fat: 25g/5 teaspoons
Oil: 60g/12 teaspoons

Spaghetti with Tomato Sauce

I have found this recipe useful for weaning youngsters off well-known brands of tinned spaghetti in tomato sauce on to slightly more interesting ways of enjoying pasta. Use long spaghetti but allow the young to have spoons and forks to cut it into short pieces before educating them in more sophisticated ways of eating this pasta.

225g/8oz spaghetti
2 cloves garlic
1 large (500g/16oz) tin tomatoes
50g/2oz grated Parmesan cheese
15ml/1 tablespoon chopped fresh parsley
2 onions
salt and pepper
30ml/2 tablespoons SFS oil
5ml/1 teaspoon basil

Cook the spaghetti for about twelve minutes in a large covered pan of boiling salted water. Heat the oil in another pan. Dice the onions and crush the garlic and cook them at a low heat in the oil until the onions are soft and golden brown. Add the tin of tomatoes, salt and pepper, parsley and basil. Simmer for about five minutes. Tip the strained spaghetti into the sauce and mix well before serving. Put the grated Parmesan in a separate dish.
Fat: 10g/2 teaspoons
Oil: 40g/8 teaspoons

Oriental Tomato Rice

225g/8oz lean leg of lamb
30ml/2 tablespoons SFS oil
1 small (225g/8oz) tin tomatoes
2 cloves garlic
2ml/½ teaspoon ground cloves
5ml/1 teaspoon ground coriander
225g/8oz long-grain rice
2ml/½ teaspoon ground cinnamon
600ml/1 pint chicken stock
1 onion
5ml/1 teaspoon salt
2ml/½ teaspoon ground ginger

Heat the oil in a pan. Dice the onion, crush the garlic and cook them in the oil until golden brown. Add the spices and stir them into the onion over the heat. Cut the meat into 25mm/1in cubes and add this to the pan, lower the heat, add the tin of tomatoes and simmer for about one hour or until the meat is tender. Add the rice, stock and salt. Bring the mixture back to the boil, cover the pan and simmer for about twenty minutes or until the rice is cooked and all the fluid is absorbed.
Fat: 20g/4 teaspoons
Oil: 40g/8 teaspoons

Risotto with Tuna Fish

30ml/2 tablespoons SFS oil
100g/4oz tinned tuna fish
1 wine glass dry white wine
600ml/1 pint water
salt and pepper
1 onion
30ml/2 tablespoons tomato puree
225g/8oz long-grain rice
½ chicken stock cube
25g/1oz grated Parmesan cheese

Dice the onion and cook it gently in the oil until it is transparent but not brown. Add the rice and stir until all the fat is absorbed. Add the tomato puree, wine, water and crumbled stock cube and bring to the boil, stirring constantly. Cover the pan, turn down the heat and simmer for about twenty minutes until the rice is cooked and all the fluid is absorbed. Drain the oil from the tuna fish, break up the fish and add it to the risotto until it has heated thoroughly. Adjust the seasoning. Serve with the Parmesan cheese.
Fat: 25g/5 teaspoons
Oil: 40g/8 teaspoons

Prawn Risotto

500g/1lb prawns
1 wine glass dry white wine
1 stalk celery
1 green pepper
125g/4oz fresh or frozen peas
1 clove garlic
salt and pepper
30ml/2 tablespoons SFS oil
1 onion
225g/8oz long-grain rice
125g/4oz button mushrooms
1 red pepper
1ml/¼ teaspoon saffron
600ml/1 pint water
chopped fresh parsley to garnish

Dice the onion and slice the peppers and celery finely. Crush the clove of garlic. Heat the oil in a thick-bottomed pan. Cook the onions, peppers and garlic until the onions are soft and transparent but not brown. Add the rice and stir until all the fat is absorbed. Add the wine and water, mushrooms, peas, saffron and seasoning. Cover the pan. Bring to the boil and simmer gently, stirring from time to time, for ten minutes. Add the prawns and simmer for

a further ten minutes. By now the rice should be tender and all the water absorbed. Serve garnished with chopped parsley.
Fat: 10g/2 teaspoons
Oil: 40g/8 teaspoons

Lasagne with Meat Sauce

225g/8oz lasagne
25g/1oz grated Parmesan cheese
salt and pepper
2 cloves garlic
225g/8oz lean minced beef
300ml/½ pint bechamel sauce
225g/8oz low-fat cottage cheese
1 egg
1 large (500g/16oz) tin tomatoes
1 onion
15ml/1 tablespoon SFS oil

For the bechamel sauce

25g/1oz PUF margarine
300ml/½ pint skimmed milk
15ml/1 tablespoon cornflour
salt and pepper

To make the bechamel sauce

Warm the margarine in a small pan, add the cornflour and stir until it is smooth. Add the milk and continue stirring until the sauce is smooth, thickened and has simmered for one minute. Season slightly.

To cook the lasagne

Bring a large uncovered pan of boiling salted water to the boil. Break each strip of lasagne into 10cm/4in lengths and cook four or five of these pieces at a time. Drop them separately into the pan of water and make sure that they have not stuck to each other once in the pan. Boil until the pieces rise to the top of the water – usually about eight minutes. Remove them, put immediately into a bowl of cold water and then spread them out on a damp cotton tea towel. Cook the rest of the lasagne in the same way.

To make the meat sauce

Heat the oil in a pan. Dice the onion, crush the garlic, add them to the oil and cook it until brown. Add the meat and stir it until it is broken up and brown. Drain off the surplus fat. Add the tin of tomatoes and salt and pepper. Cook, stirring, until the meat and tomatoes are well mixed. Put the bechamel sauce in with the meat and tomatoes and simmer uncovered for about forty minutes, stirring at frequent intervals.

To complete the dish

Put the egg and cottage cheese through an electric blender together until they are very smooth.

Place alternate layers of lasagne, meat sauce and egg-and-cottage-cheese mixture in an ovenware casserole, ending with a layer of meat sauce. Sprinkle the grated Parmesan over the top and cook in an oven at 180°C/350°F/gas mark 4 for about thirty-five minutes.

Fat: 30g/6 teaspoons
Oil: 40g/8 teaspoons

Tagliatelle with Ham and Mushrooms

350g/12oz tagliatelle
60ml/4 tablespoons dry white wine
100g/4oz lean ham
salt and pepper
100g/4oz mushrooms
15ml/1 tablespoon SFS oil
300ml/½ pint bechamel sauce (see p.118)
50g/2oz cooked peas

Boil the tagliatelle in a large covered pan of salted water for about eight minutes or less if it is home-made. Slice the mushrooms and cook gently in the oil. Add the ham, cut into narrow strips, then the wine, the peas, the bechamel sauce and the seasoning. Simmer the sauce until it is thick. Pour it over the drained tagliatelle and stir well before serving.

Fat: 10g/2 teaspoons
Oil: 20g/4 teaspoons

Jambalaya

A marvellously easy meal and, for those not on a low-fat diet, just about any sort of garlic or other sausage can be added.

45ml/3 tablespoons SFS oil
1 green pepper
2 cloves garlic
225g/8oz prawns
1 large (500g/16oz) tin tomatoes
225g/8oz long-grain rice
2ml/½ teaspoon powdered bay leaf
1ml/¼ teaspoon thyme
5ml/1 teaspoon basil
2 onions
1 red pepper
150g/6oz lean ham
150ml/¼ pint dry white wine
15ml/1 tablespoon tomato puree
15ml/1 tablespoon chopped fresh parsley
1ml/¼ teaspoon oregano
salt and pepper

Dice the onions, slice the peppers finely and crush the garlic. Cook them gently in the oil in a thick-bottomed pan until the onions are transparent. Chop the ham and add it to the pan with the prawns. Continue to cook and stir for another two to three minutes. Add the rice and stir until all the fat is absorbed. Add the tomatoes, tomato puree, wine, herbs and seasoning. Cover the pan and simmer gently for about twenty-five minutes until the rice is cooked, stirring from time to time and adding a little water if the rice is sticking.

Fat: 20g/4 teaspoons
Oil: 60g/12 teaspoons

Canneloni with Tomato Sauce

12 pieces ready-prepared canneloni
300ml/½ pint bechamel sauce (see p.118)
15ml/1 tablespoon tomato puree

For the filling

1 onion
225g/8oz minced cooked chicken
15ml/1 tablespoon SFS oil
50g/2oz mushrooms
salt and pepper

15ml/1 tablespoon flour
15ml/1 tablespoon chopped fresh parsley
1 clove garlic
1 egg
25g/1oz grated Parmesan cheese

Cook the canneloni in a large covered pan of boiling salted water, drain and leave to cool on wet greaseproof paper before filling.

Dice the onion and crush the clove of garlic and cook them gently in the oil until the onion is transparent. Add the minced chicken, chopped mushrooms, flour, parsley, seasoning and beaten egg. Stir well. Roll into long 'sausages' and feed gently into the cooled canneloni.

Stir the tomato puree into the bechamel sauce. Arrange the canneloni in an oven-proof dish. Spoon the sauce over them and sprinkle the top with grated Parmesan cheese. Cook in an oven at 190°C/375°F/gas mark 5 for about twenty minutes or until the cheese is brown.
Fat: 20g/4 teaspoons
Oil: 20g/4 teaspoons

Rice and Fish Salad

350g/12oz brown rice
90ml/6 tablespoons SFS oil
2 cloves garlic
salt and pepper
2ml/½ teaspoon saffron threads
30ml/2 tablespoons white wine vinegar
5ml/1 teaspoon dry mustard
225g/8oz cooked haddock

Cook the rice in a large pan of boiling salted water with the saffron for about thirty minutes or until the rice is tender. Drain and cool the rice. Put the oil, vinegar, garlic, mustard and seasoning in an electric blender and blend until smooth. Flake the haddock. Combine the fish and rice and toss in the dressing.
Fat: 5g/1 teaspoon
Oil: 90g/24 teaspoons

Spaghetti Bolognese

This dish is best when made with freshly prepared home-made spaghetti. Making your own pasta is time-consuming and the recipe is not, therefore, likely to be made this way often. Good Italian spaghetti can be bought or spaghetti made with wholemeal flour can be used to increase the protein content a little. The Bolognese sauce may also be used with other types of pasta. Traditionally the dish should be served sprinkled with Parmesan cheese, but the cheese can be served separately so that anybody on a low-fat diet may omit it or take a small portion.

Allow about 50g/2oz of spaghetti for each person, although more than this may be necessary for someone with a large appetite. Bring a large saucepan of water to the boil, put the ends of a handful of long spaghetti in the water and push gently into the saucepan until all the strands are submerged. Boil gently, stirring at intervals with a fork, until the spaghetti is cooked but still firm when tested between the teeth. The time will vary but will usually be between ten and fifteen minutes for ready-prepared spaghetti, less for home-made. Drain the spaghetti and keep in a warm place until you are ready to serve it. The sauce should be already cooked.

For the sauce

30ml/2 tablespoons SFS oil
1 stick celery
1 clove garlic
50g/2oz mushrooms
15ml/1 tablespoon chopped fresh parsley
salt and pepper
225g/8oz tomatoes or 1 small (225g/8oz) tin tomatoes
½ an onion
½ a medium-sized carrot
1ml/¼ teaspoon nutmeg
225g/8oz minced lean beef
7ml/½ tablespoon marjoram
90ml/6 tablespoons dry red wine

Heat the oil in a pan and gently fry the finely chopped onion, carrot, celery and crushed garlic. Turn up the heat and add the meat. Stir continuously until the meat begins to brown and sticks to the pan. Add the chopped mushrooms. Skin the tomatoes if fresh and add to the meat mixture with the wine. Boil briskly for about two minutes. Add the herbs, seasoning and nutmeg and turn down the heat. Cook very gently without a lid on the pan for about thirty-five minutes, adding a little more liquid if

necessary. The sauce should be mixed with the spaghetti before being served but if appetites vary it may be more practical to serve the sauce separately.
Fat: 20g/4 teaspoons plus Parmesan cheese if used
Oil: 40g/8 teaspoons

Chicken Pilaff

225g/8oz long-grain rice
1 onion
600ml/1 pint water
2ml/½ teaspoon ground bay leaf
2ml/½ teaspoon thyme
100g/4oz mushrooms
30ml/2 tablespoons SFS oil
2 cloves garlic
1 chicken stock cube
5ml/1 teaspoon marjoram
225g/8 oz cooked chicken cut into small pieces and with the skin removed

Dice the onion and crush the garlic. Heat the oil and cook the onion and garlic until the onion is transparent but not coloured. Add the rice and stir until all the oil is absorbed – about five minutes. Slice the mushrooms and add with all the other ingredients, making sure that the stock cube is well dissolved. Cover the pan and cook gently for about twenty minutes or until the rice is tender and all the water is absorbed.
Fat: 10g/2 teaspoons
Oil: 40g/8 teaspoons

Desserts

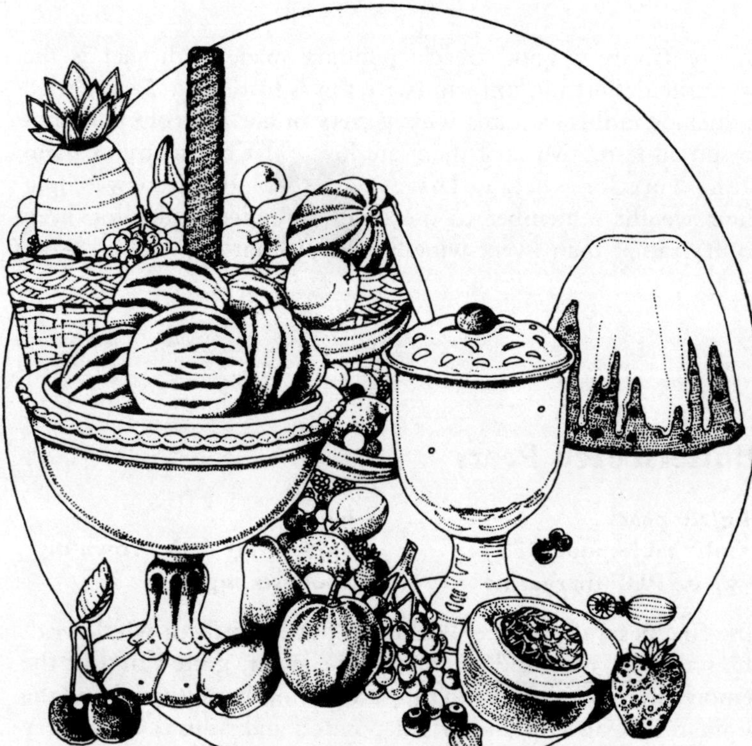

In my family a good treacle pudding made with suet is the favourite dessert but unfortunately this is forbidden. I have tried to include in this section a wide variety of hot and cold puddings to suit all tastes. Most of them are low in fat but many of them are high in calories because I have used alcohol. If you are watching your weight remember to use small amounts of alcohol, keep to dry rather than sweet wines and avoid spirits.

Butterscotch Pears

1kg/2lb pears
15ml/1 tablespoon SFS oil
25g/1oz PUF margarine
1 lemon
225g/8oz soft dark brown or molasses sugar

Use ripe pears if possible. Peel them but leave them whole with the stalks on. Heat the oil, margarine, sugar, grated rind of the lemon and lemon juice until they are a smooth mixture. Stand the pears in this sauce in an upright position and simmer them very gently until they are tender – about twenty minutes, or longer if unripe pears are used. Remove the pears and then boil the sauce without a lid until it is thick. Grasp the stalk of each pear and hold it in the syrup until liberally coated. Put the pears into a serving dish and serve them very hot or well chilled.

Fat: 5g/1 teaspoon
Oil: 40g/8 teaspoons

Caramel Ice-Cream

1 large tin sweetened skimmed condensed milk
100ml/4 fl oz warm water
2ml/½ teaspoon vanilla essence
2 eggs
50g/2oz dried skimmed milk
25g/1oz caster sugar

Put the caster sugar in a small thick-bottomed pan and watch it while it melts and turns to a warm brown colour. Do not let your attention be diverted because a burnt sugar pan takes a lot of cleaning. Whisk the dried milk in the warm water with an electric mixer until completely dissolved. Blend the tinned milk, eggs, vanilla essence and the caramelised sugar. Put it in the freezing compartment of a refrigerator or a freezer until setting round the edges. Whisk well and continue freezing.
Fat: 10g/2 teaspoons
Oil: Nil

Elderberry Sorbet

This sorbet can be made with an infusion of elderberry flowers but may also be made at any time of the year using home-made elderberry jelly for which the recipe is given on p.34.

225g/8oz elderberry jelly
50g/2oz sugar
1 egg white
300ml/½ pint water
45ml/3 tablespoons lemon juice

Dissolve the sugar in the water over a low heat and bring to the boil. Add the elderberry jelly and stir until dissolved. Add the lemon juice and leave the mixture to cool. Put it in the freezing compartment of a refrigerator or a freezer and leave it until it is freezing round the edges. Whisk the egg white until it is very stiff and whisk it gently with the freezing mixture. Whisk twice more at approximately hourly intervals and leave until of the desired consistency for serving. This will stay at a good consistency if left overnight.
Fat: Nil
Oil: Nil

Plum Water Ice

Any jam, preferably home-made, can be used for this dessert but I prefer plum or damson because it gives a tangy refreshing flavour.

500g/1lb plum or other jam
45ml/3 tablespoons lemon juice
1 egg white
450ml/¾ pint water
100g/4oz sugar

Carefully remove any stones from the plum jam and put it in an electric blender. Dissolve the sugar in the water over a low heat, bring to the boil and boil for ten minutes. Blend the syrup, jam puree and lemon juice and set aside to cool. Put in the freezing compartment of a refrigerator or freezer until freezing around the edges. Whisk the egg white until very stiff and whisk gently into the freezing mixture. Whisk at least twice more when half-frozen and then leave until of the desired consistency.
Fat: Nil
Oil: Nil

Apple and Rum Meringue

Equally good served hot or cold, but definitely for those with a sweet tooth.

For the base

50g/2oz fresh brown breadcrumbs
45ml/3 tablespoons rum

For the filling

25g/1oz PUF margarine
100g/4oz brown sugar
1kg/2lb cooking apples

For the meringue

3 egg whites
75g/3oz caster sugar
75g/3oz granulated sugar

Soak the breadcrumbs in the rum in the base of an oven-to-table

dish. Heat the margarine and brown sugar together. Add the peeled, cored and finely chopped apples. Cover and simmer gently until the apples are well cooked. I find that a potato masher will produce a coarse puree of the apples. Put the apples on the rum mixture. Whisk the egg whites until very stiff. Add half the mixed sugars and whisk gently. Add the other half and again whisk gently. Cook in an oven at 180°C/350°F/gas mark 4 for twenty-five minutes.
Fat: 5g/1 teaspoon
Oil: 40g/8 teaspoons

Figs in Wine and Honey

If you are fortunate to have a fig tree you will have no problems with this sweet. It really does need fresh figs, but should such delicacies be impossible to obtain, dried figs can be used if soaked in a little water overnight and cooked very gently.

500g/1lb fresh figs or just over half this amount of dried figs
300ml/½ pint white wine
100g/4oz honey

Place the fresh figs in a pan and cover them with wine. If you are using cooked dried figs, cook them so that all the water is absorbed and then allow them to cool before covering them with wine. Bring the figs and wine to the boil slowly and then add the honey. Chill well and serve with a mixture of cold yoghurt and skimmed-milk custard whisked together.
Fat: Nil
Oil: Nil

Banana Creams

A deliciously light and easy-to-swallow sweet – ideal for late suppers and weak digestions!

3 bananas
30ml/2 tablespoons substitute cream (see p.25)
2 egg whites
30ml/2 tablespoons home-made yoghurt
7ml/½ tablespoon caster sugar

Mash the banana until smooth. Whisk in the sugar, yoghurt and cream. Whisk the egg whites until very stiff and fold into the banana mixture. Chill in a cool place (*not* the refrigerator).
Fat: Nil
Oil: Nil

Gooseberry Sorbet

350g/12oz gooseberries
225g/8oz sugar
600ml/1 pint water
1 lemon
2 egg whites

Peel the lemon and put the strips of peel, the lemon juice, the sugar, gooseberries and water into a pan and bring them slowly to the boil. Simmer for about twenty minutes or until the gooseberries are well cooked. Remove the strips of lemon rind and put the rest of the mixture through a fine sieve. Allow this syrup to cool and then put into the freezing compartment of a refrigerator or a deep freeze and leave until it is about half-frozen. Whisk the whites of egg very stiff. Beat the frozen mixture and then beat the egg whites into it. Return to freeze and repeat the beating process at least twice more. This sweet is at its best if you allow about six hours for it to freeze or even leave it overnight.
Fat: Nil
Oil: Nil

Apricot and Orange Mousse

225g/8oz dried apricots
45ml/3 tablespoons water
100g/4oz caster sugar
juice 1 orange or 15ml/1 tablespoon unsweetened tinned orange juice
600ml/1 pint water
15g/½oz gelatine
3 egg whites

Soak the apricots in 600ml/1 pint water overnight. In the morning bring the fruit to the boil and simmer gently for about an hour or

until very soft. Dissolve the gelatine in the 45ml/3 tablespoons of cold water over a very gentle heat. Put the sugar with the hot fruit and stir until dissolved. Add the juice of an orange or 15ml/1 tablespoon unsweetened tinned orange juice. Put the fruit mixture through an electric blender until smooth. Whisk the egg whites until they are very stiff. Allow the fruit mixture to cool and fold in the egg whites. Pour into a serving dish and leave in the refrigerator until it is set.
Fat: Nil
Oil: Nil

Apple Cheesecake

For the base

75g/3oz fresh brown breadcrumbs
25g/1oz PUF margarine
25g/1oz light soft brown sugar

For the filling

500g/1lb cooking apples
50g/2oz dark soft brown sugar
250g/8oz skimmed-milk cottage cheese
1 egg
15g/½oz cornflour
50g/2oz caster sugar

Melt the margarine in a saucepan over a gentle heat and mix in the breadcrumbs and light soft brown sugar. Line an 20cm/8in flan tin with the mixture and allow it to set.

Peel, core and finely slice the cooking apples and put in a tightly covered saucepan with the soft dark brown sugar. Shake over a very gentle heat until cooking begins. Cook gently until the apples are soft and then put the mixture through a blender. Allow to cool a little and pour the apple mixture over the base in the flan tin. Put the cottage cheese, cornflour, caster sugar and the egg yolk through the blender until they are evenly mixed. Whisk the egg white stiffly and fold into the egg-yolk mixture. Pour this over the apple and cook in a moderate oven, 160°C/325°F/gas mark 3, for thirty minutes or until a pale golden colour.
Fat: 10g/2 teaspoons
Oil: Nil

Lemon Whip

300ml/½ pint cold water
2 lemons
15g/½oz gelatine
100g/4oz caster sugar
3 egg whites

Put the powdered gelatine in the cold water and leave it to soak for five minutes. Peel the rind thinly off one of the lemons and add this with the sugar and juice of both lemons to the water and gelatine. Stir over a low heat until the gelatine and the sugar have dissolved. Leave this mixture to stand in a large bowl in a cool place until it is beginning to set. Add the 3 egg whites and whisk with an electric whisk until it is thick and white. Put in a serving bowl and leave in the refrigerator until set.
Fat: Nil
Oil: Nil

Steamed Country Pudding with Brandy Sauce

When cooking or writing about puddings which are low in fat, it is all too easy to stick to fruit mousse and sorbets; but in most climates and in most families there are times when a hot pudding is much appreciated. The recipe given below is a light pudding and some or all of the whole eggs used can be substituted by the whites only.

100g/4oz currants
100g/4oz wholemeal breadcrumbs
2 whole eggs
100g/4oz finely chopped cooking apple
2ml/½ teaspoon ground nutmeg
100g/4oz raisins
30ml/2 tablespoons brandy
2 egg whites
5ml/1 teaspoon ground ginger
pinch of salt

Mix all the ingredients together and put in a well-greased bowl. Cover with foil or a double layer of greaseproof paper, secure well and steam steadily for three hours, taking care to keep the water well topped up. Turn out and serve hot with brandy sauce.

For the sauce

15ml/1 tablespoon SFS oil
15ml/1 tablespoon caster sugar
300ml/½ pint skimmed milk
15ml/1 tablespoon cornflour
30ml/2 tablespoons brandy

Warm the oil in a small saucepan. Add the cornflour and mix to a smooth consistency. Heat the prepared skimmed milk and add to the oil and flour, stirring all the time. Bring to the boil and simmer for one minute. Add the sugar and brandy. The amounts of sugar and brandy may vary according to taste.
Fat: 15g/3 teaspoons
Oil: 20g/4 teaspoons

Highland Cream

500g/1lb skimmed-milk cottage cheese
15ml/1 tablespoon bitter orange marmalade
30ml/2 tablespoons malt whisky
30ml/2 tablespoons caster sugar
15ml/1 tablespoon lemon juice

Put all the ingredients in a blender and mix until of a very smooth consistency or leave slightly uneven in texture if preferred. Put it in small ramekins and chill in the refrigerator before serving.
Fat: Nil
Oil: Nil

Sophie's Delight

I have based this sweet dessert on a recipe given me by a Chilean friend. When she no longer had servants to beat heated and sweetened milk, she found she could produce the same result by heating a tin of sweetened condensed milk in boiling water for three quarters of an hour and then cooling it before opening.

1 large tin sweetened and skimmed condensed milk
25g/1oz dried apricots
25g/1oz oatmeal
50g/2oz chopped walnuts
150ml/¼ pint dry white wine

Stand the tin of milk in a saucepan of cold water and bring it to the boil. Boil it for three quarters of an hour with the lid on. Cool and whisk with the wine. Add the chopped nuts and finely chopped apricots. Put into ramekin dishes. Brown the oatmeal lightly in a moderate oven and sprinkle over the mixture before serving.
Fat: 5g/1 teaspoon
Oil: 20g/4 teaspoons

Spiced Fruit Compôte

Various fruits can be used for this compôte. I think it is best made with a tin of black cherries, but if these are not available loganberries or strawberries are good substitutes.

150ml/¼ pint red wine
1 cinnamon stick
100g/4oz demerara sugar
500g/1lb cooking pears
425g/15oz tin black cherries or other fruit
2 ripe oranges
2 cloves

Heat the wine with the juice from the tin of fruit, the stick of cinnamon and the cloves. Bring this mixture to the boil and boil for three minutes. Add the peeled, cored and sliced pears and sugar and simmer gently until the pears are tender, adding the grated rind of the two oranges when the pears are about half-cooked. Peel the pith from the oranges. Cut the oranges into slices with a sharp knife and cut each circle across the middle. Put the oranges and the tinned fruit into a serving dish and pour the hot mixture over them. Either serve very hot or chill in the refrigerator. This dish tastes good with whipped substitute cream (see p.25).
Fat: Nil
Oil: Nil

Rhubarb and Orange Mousse

I have only discovered the delight of the combined flavours of rhubarb and orange since we moved to the north of Scotland. Fresh rhubarb is one of the few fruits grown easily, and it acquires an exotic flavour when mixed with oranges in puddings or preserves.

500g/1lb rhubarb
100g/4oz sugar
15g/½oz gelatine and 45ml/ 3 tablespoons water
50ml/2 fl oz water
1 orange
2 egg whites

Cut the rhubarb into chunks and cook gently in the 50ml/2fl oz water and sugar until tender. Grate the orange rind. Remove the skin of the orange with a sharp knife and cut the flesh into small pieces. Dissolve the gelatine in the 45ml/3 tablespoons water over a gentle heat. Put the cooked rhubarb, the grated rind and the flesh of the orange and the dissolved gelatine into a blender. Blend on a low speed. Whisk the egg whites until stiff and fold into the fruit mixture. Put in a cool place until set.
Fat: Nil
Oil: Nil

Rum Parfait

This is a delicious sweet which needs freezing overnight. It will keep well in the freezer for several days.

3 eggs
75g/3oz caster sugar
glacé fruit to decorate
100g/4oz substitute cream (see p.25)
30ml/2 tablespoons rum

Separate the egg whites and yolks. Whisk the yolks with the sugar until the mixture is light and fluffy. Add the rum and mix well. Remove the substitute cream from the freezer and whisk briefly. Mix the cream with the egg mixture. Whisk the egg whites until they are very stiff and fold them gently into the rest of the mixture. Place the dessert in a serving dish, decorate with the glacé fruit,

cover with foil and put in the freezer for a minimum of six hours but preferably overnight.
Fat: 15g/3 teaspoons
Oil: Nil

Lemon Soufflé

1 lemon
3 eggs
45ml/3 tablespoons water
125g/5oz caster sugar
100g/4oz substitute cream (see p.25)
15g/½oz gelatine

Ensure that the substitute cream is well chilled before starting to make this dish. Dissolve the gelatine in the water over a low heat. Separate the egg whites and yolks. Whisk the yolks and the sugar until they are light and fluffy. Grate the rind off the lemon and add this with the juice of the lemon to the egg mixture. Add the dissolved gelatine and whisk well. Briefly whisk the chilled substitute cream and add to the other ingredients. Whisk the egg whites until they are very stiff and fold them gently into the mixture. Put in a serving dish and leave in the refrigerator at least three hours before serving.
Fat: 15g/3 teaspoons
Oil: Nil

Pineapple Cheesecake

For the base

50g/2oz Weetabix
60ml/4 tablespoons SFS oil

For the filling

1 large tin sweetened skimmed condensed milk
225g/8oz tin crushed pineapple
225g/8oz low-fat cottage cheese
125g/5oz low-fat yoghurt
substitute cream (see p.25) for decoration
25g/1oz powdered gelatine
2 eggs
1 lemon

Warm the oil and add the crumbled Weetabix. Put the mixture into the base of a 25cm/10in diameter serving dish. Separate the eggs. Whisk the yolks of the eggs with the skimmed condensed milk. Add the grated rind of the lemon, the lemon juice and the yoghurt and whisk again. Dissolve the gelatine in the juice from the tin of crushed pineapple over a gentle heat and whisk into the egg mixture. Put the cottage cheese into a blender and mix until very smooth. Add the crushed pineapple and blend until of the required consistency. Add the cheese and pineapple to the egg mixture and whisk for a further thirty seconds. Whisk the egg whites until very stiff and fold into the mixture, pour over the prepared base and allow to set in the refrigerator – about three hours. Decorate with the substitute cream.

Fat: 10g/2 teaspoons
Oil: 40g/8 teaspoons

Black Cherry Cheesecake

For the base

50g/2oz Weetabix
15ml/1 tablespoon soft brown sugar
60ml/4 tablespoons SFS oil

For the filling

1 tin black cherry pie-filling
125g/5oz low-fat yoghurt
225g/8oz low-fat cottage cheese
45ml/3 tablespoons water
15g/½oz cornflour
100g/4oz substitute cream (see p.25)
15g/½oz gelatine

Make the base by mixing the warmed fat with the crumbled Weetabix and sugar and press firmly into an 20cm/8in flan dish. Dissolve the gelatine in the water over a low heat. Put the cottage cheese in a blender to make the consistency very fine. Mix the cottage cheese, yoghurt, gelatine and cream substitute together and whisk for a minute. Place the mixture on the flan base and leave in a refrigerator to set.

Mix the cornflour with a tablespoon of the pie filling to a

smooth consistency and add the remainder of the black cherry pie-filling. Bring the mixture to the boil and allow to simmer for one minute. Allow to cool a little and then spread over the flan.
Flan: Nil
Oil: 40g/8 teaspoons

Fruit Pavlova

Any fresh or frozen fruit may be used but good fresh strawberries are always my favourites. I have made this recipe with frozen strawberries but it is better to allow them to thaw slowly and put the fruit on the cream substitute immediately before serving.

4 egg whites
5ml/1 teaspoon cornflour
225g/8oz whipped substitute cream (see p.25)
225g/8oz caster sugar
5ml/1 teaspoon lemon juice
fresh fruit of your choice

Beat the egg whites until very stiff. Add half the sugar and beat again slowly. Add the remainder of the sugar and beat again. Finally add the cornflour and lemon juice and beat again briefly. Wring out a large sheet of greaseproof paper in cold water and put it on a wire tray. Spread the meringue mixture over this in a circle and bake in an oven at 130°C/250°F/gas mark ½ for about two hours until it is crisp. Allow to cool. Spread liberally with the *lightly* whipped cream and top with fruit immediately before serving.
Fat: Nil
Oil: Nil

Chilled Raspberry Soufflé

225g/8oz fresh or frozen raspberries
15g/½oz gelatine
30ml/2 tablespoons water
3 egg whites
50g/2oz caster sugar
30ml/2 tablespoons redcurrant jelly
100g/4oz whipped substitute cream (see p.25)

Warm the raspberries and the sugar in the top of a double cooker until the sugar has dissolved and the raspberries are very soft. Put the fruit mixture through a fine sieve. Dissolve the gelatine in the redcurrant jelly and water over a low heat and mix thoroughly with the raspberry mixture. Allow this to cool. Add the whipped cream. Beat the egg whites until they are very stiff and fold gently into the rest of the sweet. Put into a serving dish and leave in the refrigerator for several hours before serving.
Fat: Nil
Oil: Nil

Baked Syrup Pie

3 Weetabix
1 large cooking apple
30ml/2 tablespoons golden syrup
75g/3oz fresh breadcrumbs
15ml/1 tablespoon PUF margarine
30ml/2 tablespoons skimmed milk
1 lemon
5ml/1 teaspoon cinnamon
15ml/1 tablespoon soft dark brown sugar

Crush the Weetabix in a blender and warm gently in a saucepan with the margarine. Put the mixture in the base of an 20cm/8in flan tin, and press down firmly. Peel, core and grate the cooking apple. Add the apple to the breadcrumbs, golden syrup, grated rind and juice of the lemon and milk and heat gently until well mixed. Spread evenly over the base in the flan tin. Sprinkle the dark brown sugar and cinnamon evenly over the top and bake in a moderate oven for about thirty minutes at 180°C/350°F/gas mark 4.
Fat: 2·5g/½ teaspoon
Oil: 10g/2 teaspoons

Scones and Cakes

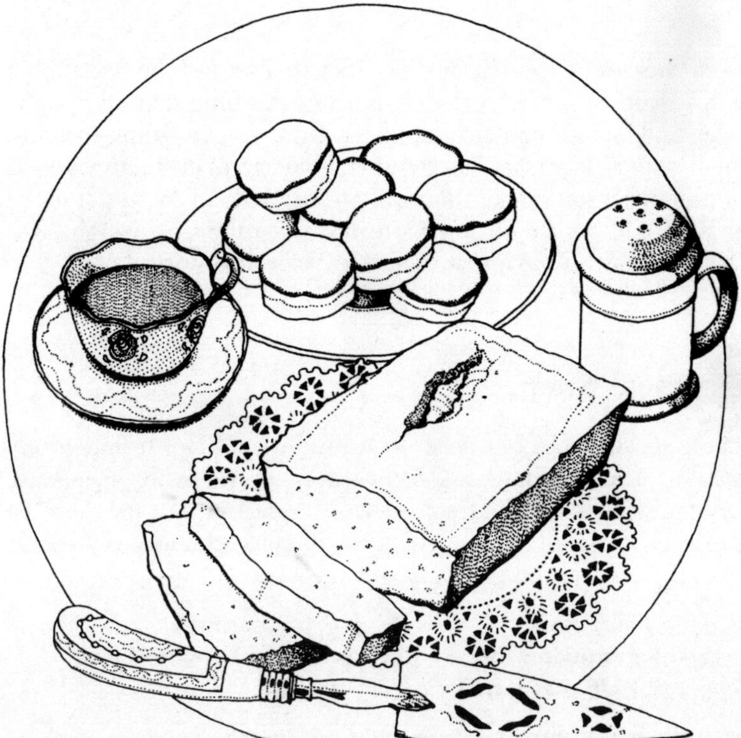

Even those on a low-fat diet like their snacks and the odd nibble with a cup of tea or coffee. It is safe to assume that all bought cakes and biscuits contain animal fat and if you are going to enjoy them with a clear conscience you will have to make them yourself or preferably get one of the family to make them for you. I make no apologies for the strong Scottish streak running through these recipes; Scottish baking at its best is second to none.

Oatmeal Snaps

These are delicious but need great care in cooking. If underdone they are tooth-pulling; and if overdone they readily incinerate. My family will eat the results even if imperfect, but these can be denture-snapping! When perfect the biscuits seldom survive long enough to be stored in an airtight tin.

75g/3oz plain flour
125g/5oz granulated sugar
100g/4oz PUF margarine
75g/3oz oatmeal
30ml/2 tablespoons black treacle

Melt the margarine, the sugar and the treacle together over a low heat, stirring constantly. Add the dry ingredients. Put small teaspoonsful on to a well-greased baking sheet, spaced well apart. Bake at 180°C/350°F/gas mark 4 for six to ten minutes but *watch carefully*. Remove from the oven, leave to cool a little and then lift off the baking sheet with a cake-slice or sharp knife.
Fat: 20g/4 teaspoons
Oil: 80g/16 teaspoons

Swiss Nutty Biscuits

Like many sweet nutty recipes, these are best for those with sound teeth, but they are delicious.

100g/4oz ground brazil nuts
50g/2oz sugar
25g/1oz flour
15ml/1 tablespoon honey
100g/4oz ground walnuts
1 egg white
15ml/1 tablespoon brandy
2ml/½ teaspoon mixed spice

Beat the egg white until it is beginning to thicken. Warm the honey and then mix all the ingredients together. Flatten on a board with your lightly floured hand and cut into strips about 25 × 50mm/1 × 2in. Cook on a greased baking tin in a slow oven, 150°C/300°F/gas mark 2, for about twenty minutes. Watch the biscuits carefully and remove from the oven while they are still soft. Leave to dry on a rack before storing.
Fat: 50g/10 teaspoons
Oil: 60g/12 teaspoons

Orkney Gingerbread

75g/3oz PUF margarine
150g/6oz oatmeal
10ml/2 teaspoons baking powder
5ml/1 teaspoon ground ginger
1 egg
150g/6oz wholemeal flour
100g/4oz sugar
300ml/½ pint skimmed milk
30ml/2 tablespoons black treacle

Put the treacle, margarine, sugar and egg together in a pan and warm them stirring gently until they are soft and well mixed. Add the flour, sifted with the baking powder, and half the milk. Stir well. Add the ginger and oatmeal and enough of the other half of the milk to make a mixture that will drop easily from a spoon. Put in a greased square or oblong tin and bake in a moderate oven, 180°C/350°F/gas mark 4, for about one hour until it is well risen and spongy to the touch. It is best, but in our house impossible, to leave the gingerbread for twenty-four hours before cutting it.
Fat: 20g/4 teaspoons
Oil: 60g/12 teaspoons

Date and Treacle Cake

225g/8oz flour
50g/2oz sugar
150g/6oz chopped dates
30ml/2 tablespoons water
5ml/1 teaspoon mixed spice
5ml/1 teaspoon baking powder
50g/2oz PUF margarine
60ml/4 tablespoons black treacle
1 egg
45ml/3 tablespoons skimmed milk

Rub the fat into the flour and baking powder. Add the dates with the sugar, mixed spice, lightly beaten egg, treacle, water and skimmed milk. Mix to a stiff consistency and bake in a greased bread tin in a moderate oven, 180°/350°F/gas mark 4, for one hour. Turn on to a rack and cool.
Fat: 15g/3 teaspoons
Oil: 40g/8 teaspoons

Treacle Scones

225g/8oz flour
2ml/½ teaspoon baking powder
2ml/½ teaspoon cream of tartar
30ml/2 tablespoons melted treacle
skimmed milk to mix
2ml/½ teaspoon salt
25g/1oz PUF margarine
50g/2oz caster sugar
5ml/1 teaspoon mixed spice

Mix the dry ingredients together. Rub in the margarine. Add the treacle and enough milk to make a soft elastic dough. Roll out the dough to a thickness of 12mm/½in. Cut into circles about the size of a saucer and bake on a hot oiled girdle until well risen and brown on both sides. Alternatively, bake in a hot oven, 200°C/400°F/gas mark 6, for about ten minutes.
Fat: 5g/1 teaspoon
Oil: 20g/4 teaspoons

Oatmeal Scones

150g/6oz flour
10ml/2 teaspoons baking powder
1ml/¼ teaspoon salt
50g/2oz oatmeal
50g/2oz PUF margarine
skimmed milk to mix

Mix the dry ingredients together, rub in the margarine and mix to a soft dough with the skimmed milk. Roll out until the dough is about 12mm/½in thick. Cut it into rounds and bake the scones in a hot oven, 220°C/425°F/gas mark 6, for about ten minutes. Cool on a wire tray.
Fat: 10g/2 teaspoons
Oil: 40g/8 teaspoons

Butterscotch Brownies

Delicious but fattening. Be very careful not to overcook them.

75g/3oz PUF margarine
1 egg
1ml/¼ teaspoon salt
2ml/½ teaspoon vanilla essence
125g/5oz soft dark brown sugar
75g/3oz wholemeal flour
7ml/1½ teaspoons baking powder
50g/2oz chopped walnuts

Melt the margarine and sugar together and add all the other ingredients. Put into a greased 20cm/8in square tin and bake in a moderate oven, 180°C/350°F/gas mark 4, for about thirty minutes. Remove the brownies from the oven before they begin to darken round the outside and shrink away from the side of the tin. Cut into sixteen squares while hot. Allow to cool a little, then remove from the tin and put on a rack to cool.
Fat: 25g/5 teaspoons
Oil: 80g/16 teaspoons

Spicy Biscuits

175g/7oz flour
75g/3oz soft dark brown sugar
5ml/1 teaspoon mixed spice
1 egg
5ml/1 teaspoon baking powder
75g/3oz ground hazelnuts
100g/4oz PUF margarine

Mix all the ingredients together on a floured board and work into a dough. Break off small pieces, roll them into balls and then flatten them a little. Put them on a greased baking tin and bake in moderately hot oven, 190°C/375°F/gas mark 5, for about ten minutes.
Fat: 50g/10 teaspoons
Oil: Nil

Melting Moments

25g/1oz PUF margarine
60ml/4 tablespoons SFS oil
150g/6oz flour
100g/4oz caster sugar
2ml/½ teaspoon vanilla essence
5ml/1 teaspoon baking powder

Cream the margarine and sugar together until fluffy – a hand beater is very useful for this. Add the oil gradually and beat thoroughly. Add the vanilla, flour and baking powder to form a dough. Roll the dough into small balls and put them on a greased baking tin. Bake for about fifteen minutes in a moderately hot oven, 180°C/350°F/gas mark 4.
Fat: 5g/1 teaspoon
Oil: 100g/20 teaspoons

Macaroons

100g/4oz ground almonds
1ml/¼ teaspoon almond essence
75g/3oz icing sugar
1 egg white

Beat together all the ingredients until a smooth dough is formed. Roll the dough into small balls and bake them on oiled greaseproof paper in a hot oven, 220°C/425°F/gas mark 7, for about six minutes until they are golden in colour but still spongy to touch.
Fat: 40g/8 teaspoons
Oil: 10g/2 teaspoons

Bere Meal Scones

100g/4oz flour
10ml/2 teaspoons baking powder
150ml/¼ pint skimmed milk
100g/4oz bere or barley meal
50g/2oz PUF margarine
2ml/½ teaspoon salt

Sieve the flour with the salt and baking powder. Mix in the bere meal. Rub in the margarine and mix to a dough with the milk. Roll out 12mm/½in thick and cut into saucer-sized circles. Score each circle across twice to make marks for four scones. Bake in a hot oven, 220°C/425°F/gas mark 7, for ten minutes. Cool on a wire tray.
Fat: 10g/2 teaspoons
Oil: 40g/8 teaspoons

Honey Bread

This quantity is enough for two loaves.

350g/12oz wholemeal flour
10ml/2 teaspoons baking powder
50g/2oz PUF margarine
150g/6oz clear honey
150ml/¼ pint water
2ml/½ teaspoon salt
5ml/1 teaspoon mixed spice
150g/6oz demerara sugar
1 egg
100g/4oz currants

Sieve all the dry ingredients together. Rub in the margarine and add the sugar, fruit, beaten egg and honey. Mix very well with the water. Put the mixture in two greased loaf tins and bake in a moderate oven, 180°C/350°F/gas mark 4, for about one hour.
Fat: 10g/2 teaspoons
Oil: 40g/8 teaspoons

Index